Doctor, Have you got a minute?

Doctor, Have you got a minute?

Dr Tom Smith

✳ SHORT BOOKS

First published in 2006 by
Short Books
3A Exmouth House, Pine Street
London EC1R OJH
10 9 8 7 6 5 4 3 2 1
Copyright ©
Tom Smith 2006

A CIP catalogue record for this book
is available from the British Library.

Jacket design © James Nunn 2006
Jacket illustration © Lesley Anderson 2006

ISBN 1-904977- 79-0
(978-1-904977-79-7)
Printed and bound in Great Britain by
William Clowes Ltd, Beccles, Suffolk

For my family

Introduction

I've thought about writing this book for nearly a quarter of a century. That's how long I've been answering questions in my doctor column in various newspapers. Most of the questions I receive from readers are fairly predictable, even dull, but many are, shall we say, unusual. They are the sort that can't be answered by looking up the journals, and wouldn't be asked in a routine surgery appointment. So this isn't the usual collection of questions and answers that you would read in any doctor's column in a newspaper. They are, I suppose, a mixture of the sort of questions I've been asked socially, often at dinner parties, and especially towards the end of the evening. They take in the quirky, the funny, and sometimes the serious.

Answering medical questions outside the surgery

environment, whether it's at a party or at the bus stop, is 'off the top of your head' stuff. Unlike 'real' medicine in the surgery, there's no instant access to the books and journals, or to the internet, to give doctors the chapter and verse back-up to what we are saying. Nor do we have the opportunity to take a proper history, examine the patient and set up tests to prove the diagnosis – all essentials in every surgery consultation. So when we pontificate socially on a subject we rely on our experience and what we remember about what we have read.

Consequently, I have to admit that this book is flawed. I have answered queries very much as I would do in every day life: ie, pretty much 'off the cuff'. This has the advantage that, while reading it, you won't be bothered by footnotes or by references to obscure reports in magazines you haven't heard of, and I get to write freely and in my own completely biased way about the medical world as I see it.

That said, I'm fairly certain that what I write is accurate for its time: every week I read the *British Medical Journal*, the *Lancet* and the *New Scientist*, mostly from cover to cover. And then there is what I've heard.

For around a quarter of a century I have been reporting medical conferences all round the world. It is like being paid to be a permanent student of medicine. So when I'm asked, for example, at a drinks party, about the health benefits of red wine, I can say I was there, in Paris (or was it Vienna? That's memory for you), when they were first announced.

Conversations with a doctor you have only just met are hardly the best for rational and sympathetic discussion, of course, and are rarely as fruitful as they may seem on the night. With the morning hangover (possibly for both participants) comes the realisation that what was said the previous evening might have been better left unsaid. For the doctor that's especially so when the person's real doctor phones up, irate about interference with the precious doctor-patient relationship, and threatens to report the apparently drunken conversation to the disciplinary committee of the General Medical Council. Suffice to say, if you are seriously worried about something, you should visit your own GP. Here I merely offer some of the commonest, and oddest, questions that I have been asked over the years. Perhaps you'll recognise yourself in one of the types...

The Beauty Junky

Who is happy with their shape and appearance? Apparently about 80 per cent of men don't really care, and about the same number of women hate how they look and would like to change themselves. At least that's what the magazines would have us believe. I'm not sure it's true. Most of the young women I know seem to be happy with themselves, and that doesn't seem to change when they grow older.

And then there's the Beauty Junky. She stalks the earth looking for ways to improve her appearance. She's not happy with her skin, her nose, her bust, her spots, her figure, her posture, her hair, her laughter lines (when did you ever hear a Beauty Junky call her wrinkles that?) or, in fact, her life. So she tries to improve them all with creams, with fancy diets, with pills – mostly vitamins, supplements and herbs – and eventually with botox and surgery.

She talks about hardly anything other than ways to keep herself looking young – plastic surgery, collagen, botox and the like – and is most exercised by a material called cellulite, unknown to medical science, that has mysteriously appeared under the skin of her thighs. Currently she is trying to eradicate this material by slapping it with a vibrating belt and beating it with birch twigs in a sauna. She isn't having much success.

Thankfully she disappears every now and then from the social scene, to recover from her latest nose or boob job, but afterwards she is back again with renewed enthusiasm and a face that is even more devoid of expression.

She is probably the most frustrating of all the people who plague doctors. Not for her the evidence of clinical trials and of disastrous case histories: she would rather believe the ads of the very wealthy (and often unscrupulous) companies that promote their beauty products. I often wonder, while the Beauty Junky is prattling on about her next adventure in the search for eternal beauty and perfect health, if she has ever read Rider Haggard's *She*. (The eternally youthful heroine visited the rejuvenating flame once too often, with terrible results.) But, of course, I'm too polite to ask.

Will I age at the same rate as my mother?

It depends a lot on whether your life and lifestyle have mirrored hers. They probably haven't. You probably grew up in better conditions, ate better, had fewer health knocks in your life, and had an altogether more affluent lifestyle. In which case you will age more slowly than your mother. The biggest influence on ageing in our society, however, is smoking. Smoking rapidly accelerates the ageing process. So if your mother was a non-smoker and you smoke, despite all your other advantages, you will age much faster than she did. It's not just the wrinkles, but the effects that smoking, carbon monoxide and tars have on all the internal organs, too. Smokers' lungs can sometimes seem 40 years older than their owner actually is.

Is it true that some people have better metabolisms than others? Or can you be fat while not eating very much?

No, people don't have different metabolisms. Our basic human metabolism is universally very similar: if it does differ in its rate it is almost always because of an illness, like thyroid gland disease (either over- or under-activity). And yes, you can be fat while not eating very much.

Let's go back to studies of 'fidgets and floppers' done around 40 years ago. Volunteers were put in 'calorie-controlled' rooms for a few days. Everything in the room was constantly measured – the heat the people gave off, their physical activity, the material they expelled (for want of a better phrase) and their weights on entry and leaving several days later. The food intake was controlled so that everyone ate the same each day. The temperature of each room was kept constant, at a comfortable level. At the end, half of the subjects had kept to the same weight; the others had put on several kilos.

The difference between them? The steady weight people had never been still. Even when they were sitting down, they were moving their fingers, their limbs, shifting in their seats, and getting up and down a lot. They were the 'fidgets'. The weight gainers tended to flop in a chair and not move out of it until the food was pushed through the hatch in the wall. They hardly ever got up and walked around. When they were seated, they hardly moved a muscle. They flopped and stayed flopped.

Now turn to the Danes in 2005. The Danes are a great help in answering questions like this. They have a captive population – the whole country, whose medical records are on the same database. They followed all the children born in Denmark in a single year from their ninth birthdays until they were 18. They watched their food consumption, their weight gain, their body shapes and the amount of exercise they took over their teenage years. About 15 per cent of them became obese in that time. What had made them obese? Not their food intake. On average, the slim Danes had eaten the same food as the fat ones. The big difference was in their exercise. The slim ones rode bicycles to school and played games and sports a lot. The fatter ones rode in their parents' cars or the bus to school and preferred video games at home to the outdoors. So you can be fat while not overeating. The big difficulty for some people is to rustle up enough energy to burn off the fat.

Does that mean that the only way we can lose weight is to exercise, and that dieting doesn't work?

Oh, no it doesn't. We BECOME fat by not exercising, but we STAY fat and get fatter by eating too much, as well as being couch potatoes. So we must both cut down on what we eat and exercise more.

So what's the best way to cut down? I've tried every diet there is and I am still not thin.

The best answer is to eat more slowly. The feeling that you are hungry takes a while to die down even when you are stuffing your mouth and stomach with food. If you eat fast, you will get a lot more food inside you before you feel satisfied than if you eat more slowly. The old Victorians were right – they taught children to put small amounts of food into their mouths at a time, then chew it 32 times before swallowing it.

Maybe in their time, when everyone had such rotten teeth (why do you think those country houses had so many jelly moulds in their kitchens?), chewing was a laborious and inefficient business, and it took longer than it does today to chew solid food until it was in a fit state to swallow.

Be that as it may, take some time to chew each mouthful of food before swallowing it: 32 times is pretty excessive – but do enjoy the tastes, savour the last swallow before picking up the fork again for the next mouthful, and make its size half of what you used to put on a fork. If you can draw out the first part of your meal for 25 minutes, even if you have eaten only a fraction of your usual by this time, you will feel much less hungry. You won't want to eat loads for the next course, and will probably do without a dessert altogether. At least that is what you should aim for. The method works, and it has the benefits that you can eat and enjoy all the foods you like, and even enjoy the fact that you are eating less. The

French and Italians have the right idea – they make eating a family affair, in which the act of eating is only part of the entertainment. There's drinking, conversation, fun, music and sociability that makes eating an occasion. They eat and drink less over four hours than we Brits do in one. For the proof of my argument go to Paris for a day and look at the Parisians. Then return to any British city and look at the people in the streets. Which has the biggest proportion of blobbies? I rest my case.

Why is one breast bigger than the other – and does it relate to whether you are right- or left-handed?

We aren't designed to be exactly symmetrical. Look at the two halves of your face. Split your face down the middle, make a mirror image of each half, stick the mirror images together and you will see two people who vaguely look like you, and who look even less like each other. It's similar for breasts – we can't expect the breast on one side of the chest to grow to be exactly the same as the other one. They can differ in volume by around a third. Which one is the bigger is decided simply by chance. The question of whether or not breast size is linked to handedness presumably arises from the bulk of the chest muscles underneath each breast. As those on the side of the dominant hand are slightly bigger (but not noticeably so), in a right-handed woman the right breast might be expected to be more prominent. There's no evidence that it is. Handedness can have no influence on the size of the breast tissue itself.

Why do women grow beards?

Part of this may be due to a subtle change in circulating hormone levels, as the normal ratio of oestrogen to progesterone (the two main female sex hormones) changes. The more progesterone and the less oestrogen you have, the more likely you are to become hairy. There's also the masculinising effect of a constant production of testosterone, which isn't exclusive to males, and which doesn't fall with age in women, so that its relative influence is greater. Testosterone underlies the female libido – the higher your testosterone level the greater your sex urge. It's unfortunate that this coincides with the appearance of a hairy chin.

Why are some people more moley than others?

We humans display an amazing range of skin colouring,

from the Scandinavian's very light skin to the blackest skin of the African equatorial regions, and every shade in between. The colour depends on the amount of the pigment melanin in the skin – the blacker the skin is, the more melanin we have deposited in it. In some people with lighter skin, the melanin cells, instead of being uniformly distributed throughout, are left in 'patches'. They may have 200 or more moles, often in lines, mainly on their backs. The lighter the rest of your skin, the more moles you are likely to have. Black-skinned people have very few moles. The tendency to have a lot of moles (several hundreds) is inherited. If you have them, you should check on them regularly (a partner is helpful if they are on your back) because there is a small but definite increased risk of change towards cancer as you age, especially if you have exposed them regularly to the sun.

Is it true that food eaten on an aeroplane does not make you put on weight?

Of course it isn't. Does getting on an aeroplane suspend the fundamental laws of physics? Or medicine? No. Food eaten on an aeroplane has exactly the same effect on your weight as food on the ground. The fact that you are eating it at a relative altitude of around 8,000 feet (the air pressure inside a plane is set as equivalent to that height) makes no difference. Mind you, maybe the quality of the food has to be taken into account: I'm not sure there were any calories in the stuff I was given on my last shuttle flight between Glasgow and Heathrow.

Do we really need pubic hair? I seem to spend my life removing it.

Do cars need shock absorbers? Do the pelvic skin and bone under the hair not need protection from another pelvic bone banging or grinding against them? Try having energetic sex with both pubic areas shaved and that might provide your answer. I don't recommend it myself, but then I'm probably a grumpy old fuddy-duddy born in the years before sex was invented.

How long do the effects of cosmetic surgery, such as wrinkle removal, last? Does it have to be renewed after a time?

If you are thinking of botox injections, then between three and six months. At which point the muscles that have been paralysed by this enormously powerful poison return, and with them the wrinkles. If you are thinking of surgical removal of wrinkles, such as those on a turkey neck, then maybe the appearance will last a year or two longer. Much depends on how you acquired the wrinkles in the first place. If you are a smoker, for example, then they will come back a lot faster, as the chemicals in the smoke begin to destroy the skin again.

Why is it that my laser eye surgeon wears glasses – does he know something I don't?

Good question. Yes he does. He knows that up to 5 per cent of people who have laser surgery can't see all that well afterwards – they have permanently blurred vision that isn't fully corrected by glasses.

There are two essential requirements of a consultant eye surgeon. One is that he is good at his job. The other is that he can see perfectly, so that he can do his job. Would you take any risk with your eyesight if you were an eye surgeon? Most people can get away with slightly impaired vision – in fact, most people do. That's why there's such a queue for laser surgery. But surgeons can't. I don't mind wearing glasses: I've worn them since I was a student. I'd be lost without them, but with them I can see perfectly enough to watch a small white ball fly about 200 yards from my club deep into gorse. As long as I can still do that with my specs, I don't want laser surgery.

Do we age faster if we work in an air-conditioned environment?

No we don't. You may be thinking of your skin being constantly dehydrated, but drinking plenty of water is enough to keep you crease-free. Good air-conditioning should give you air that is as healthy as any unpolluted atmosphere outside. However, if this air-conditioned environment is an office which keeps you tied to your desk with no opportunity for regular exercise, that can make you age faster.

Is cholesterol something only men should worry about?

You would think this is an easy question to answer, but it isn't. Almost all the research has been done in men: the equivalent women's studies are still ongoing. For men the answer is straightforward. The total cholesterol is best kept under 5.2 units (under our system in the UK the units are millimoles per litre), and the ratio of total cholesterol to high-density cholesterol (HDL) should be under 5:1.

That probably sounds obscure to you, but HDL is the 'good' cholesterol, the substance that clears fats out of our blood vessel walls, The other two main substances that make up the total cholesterol are 'bad' lipids that tend to deposit fats into them. They are LDL or low-density cholesterol (the L stands for lipoprotein, a complex of fat and protein), and VLDL (very low-density lipoprotein, or triglycerides). Add the three together, and you get the total cholesterol.

Got it so far? To judge whether or not you are at high risk, the crucial measurement is the ratio between the HDL cholesterol and the total cholesterol. If HDL forms more than one-fifth of the total, then there is little need to worry about it. So a total cholesterol of, say, 7 is fine if the HDL is around 3, but not if it is around 1.

The higher the cholesterol readings, the greater the risk you run of a heart attack and stroke – since we started to concentrate on reducing cholesterol levels in British men we have reduced their stroke and heart attack rates by around a half. This is a fantastic achievement.

So it's not looking great for women?

Before we started measuring and treating cholesterol

levels, the women's risks of heart attacks and strokes rose with age in the same way as men's – except 10 years later than them. So the average 60-year-old man's chances of a heart attack were the same as those of a 70-year-old woman. This was good news for the females. There's some suggestion that their relative resistance to heart attacks and strokes is due to the protective effect that the female hormones exert on blood vessels during their menstrual years.

These figures have tended to make doctors regard cholesterol levels in women as less important than those in men. But there are several problems with that. Women who smoke, have poorly controlled high blood pressure, and who have been on HRT for more than six months, are all at higher risk of heart attack and stroke than other women. If they want to improve their health, it's suggested that they stop smoking, have their blood pressure regularly monitored and controlled, stop their HRT *and* have their cholesterol lowered if it is above the limits set for men. We do that routinely today as doctors, and it probably works.

So how do we reconcile this practice with the result of French studies which showed that the average cholesterol in women over 80 years old is above 8 millimoles per litre? Maybe French women are different. Maybe their cholesterol levels have increased with age (though that doesn't seem to have happened elsewhere) or maybe all the women with lower cholesterol levels have died off before they reached 80? It is possible that, for some women, high cholesterol is good. We don't know yet.

On the whole, I still tend to try to lower cholesterol levels in women in whom they are too high, but it is a low priority, to be tackled after I have dealt with their other 'heart' risks. Smoking and uncontrolled high blood pressure kill far more women than does high cholesterol.

Can repeatedly dyeing your hair cause it to fall out?

There's evidence that some dyes can kill off hair follicles, at least in animal studies. You seem to need a combination of hydrogen peroxide, amines and phenols for them to do so, so if you want to keep a thick head of hair, avoid dyes that contain these chemicals. It's curious that people having regular hair dyes hardly ever ask to see their ingredients. When did you last do so? You would want to know what you were swallowing if it were a food or a medicine – and hair dyes are in contact with the scalp, which can certainly absorb their ingredients. If you are worried, what about staying grey and calling your hair silver? It could be your fashion statement.

Does jogging harm your knees?

It shouldn't hurt normal knees if you choose the correct footwear, with cushioning under the soles and heels. But for people who already have knees with damaged cartilages or the beginnings of arthritis, it may make things worse. If your knees begin to hurt during and after jogging, see your doctor about it. You may have to choose another form of exercise. Brisk walking is just as good for you. Swimming's OK too, but you may find breaststroke a bit difficult. Crawl and backstroke are probably better for you if your knees are dodgy.

The Mid-Life Male

The Germans have a great name for what this guy has – the *'tur-schluss* complex'. I hope my German is correct, forgive me if it isn't. Obviously, it means the door-shutting complex. The Mid-life Male is realising that the door is shutting on his youth (or even middle age) and he wants to grab as much as life can offer him before he slides down the other side of the razor blade of life to eventual oblivion. Dare I mention certain eminent politicians in this context?

The first sign that a man has become a mid-life male is that he has started to dress differently: flashy ties and shirts have replaced the more sober ones he favoured in his thirties. Out go the business suits and in come the motorbike, the bomber jackets and glossy shoes. He is worried about his potency (he wants to retain it); his hair (ditto); and his middle-aged spread (he wants to lose this, but not by eating or drinking less). He is only just finding out that all these ambitions are beyond his reach.

He has started to exercise again, having stopped when he left school around 20 years ago. Now he has joined the local gym (one with plenty of female customers), the five-a-side football team and the local running club. He is killing himself with over-exercise in trying to stay young, and he wants all the hints on how he can do so. His conversation revolves around cholesterol levels, blood pressure, heart attacks and sex. In a few years, if he survives this terrible decade, he will settle down to a normal life again, and become almost human.

Why do men, and not women, go bald?

Let's take you back to around 12 million years ago when our ancestors were still small ape-like creatures stumbling around scratching a living in the forests of East Africa – what is now Kenya. The climate changed suddenly, and the forested plain was transformed within a few hundred years into a grassy plain. Our small apes now had a choice to make. Either they followed the receding tree line up into the hills, where they became the chimpanzees, or they fled the other way, to the coast.

There they could survive only in the lagoons between beach and reef, where they were protected from the big cats and, by the reef, from the big sharks.

It was idyllic. For eight million years, the apes stayed in the lagoons. They became taller, developed hands and feet like oars and paddles, lost almost all their body hair so that they could swim better, and developed the necessary layer of fat under the skin to keep their body heat at the optimum. The nose developed nostrils that would prevent water entering it. The legs even started to grow together, as they were on the way to becoming fully aquatic (that's why our genitalia moved forwards, to accommodate the movement of thighs towards each other). The problem came for the babies. What were they to hold on to in this watery environment when there was danger, or when they wanted to breast-feed?

The best thing was long hair. Mothers who kept the hair on top of their heads were easy to recognise and offered a good handhold for baby. So the gene for baldness in women died out. However there was no point in father keeping his hair, as he didn't have functioning breasts. In the survival of the fittest, baldness put men at no particular disadvantage, so the baldness gene had no reason to die out.

Then, after eight million years in the lagoons, the apes returned to the land. They were much better able to fend for themselves, as they were now socially well-knit in families. They were twice the height they had been eight million years before, had a bigger brain, and they could oversee any predator, now that their eyes were three feet or so higher off the ground. They were very far away now from their cousins that had opted for the hill forests eight million years before.

Sounds improbable? All this is the theory of Elaine Morgan, the distinguished Welsh anthropologist. As a Scot I like to give credit to a fellow Celt – but she didn't at first get any credit for her work. She wrote *The Descent of Woman* partly as a response to *The Ascent of Man* written by the Seventies TV guru Jacob Bronowski, and partly to put her research in the public eye. The mostly male anthropological establishment of the time gave her short shrift, but today she is held in high esteem, and her theory of the time our ancestors spent in the shallows of East Africa is accepted by many of her peers.

It may resolve a lot of puzzles over and above the baldness question. It could explain, for example, why we humans are so at home in water, enjoy swimming and beach holidays, and why the vast majority of human communities are on coasts or at least in near reach of seas and rivers. It may also explain why we still have pubic hair – babies can grab on to that, too. And what about that hand-penis relationship? (See the next question.) Well, the hands were developing into paddles to get us through the water. The bigger the paddles, the more efficient we were,

34

and therefore the more manly we were. Does that relate to penis size, too? Or does size really matter that much? Our modern women are not so concerned. Its main function is to reach their G-spot: it doesn't need to be very long to do that.

There is a postscript to the baldness question. Of course, some women do go bald, but it is rare for them to do so before the menopause – and the gene that allows post-menopausal baldness would not have prevented successful motherhood in our lagoon-living ancestors. But they are a very small minority of women. When a younger woman does go bald, their doctors have to rule out physical causes, such as scalp infections or alopecia.

I remember here with much affection a woman in her early forties with two children who asked my advice on her baldness. It had started around two years before, and was now almost total, with hair only around the tops of her ears and around the back of her head. To my shock, the dermatologist diagnosed male-pattern baldness, and ordered, secretly (this could be done at the time), genetic tests. It turned out that this woman was in fact a true male, with female external genitals and testes that were inside her pelvis, producing a mixture of testosterone and oestrogen. There was no womb, but she did have a functioning vagina.

She was a perfectly feminine woman, brought up as a woman, who, apart from her baldness (for which we arranged an excellent wig), looked very attractive. Her husband and children (who had been adopted – something I learned only after the diagnosis) adored her. So what were we to do? The dermatologist and I decided not to tell anyone – a decision that probably could not have been taken today.

The couple lived happily on into retirement and died ignorant of her true status. In all the time I have been a family doctor, this was my only case of such a gender mix-up. I'm not sure that it adds support to Dr Morgan's theory, but it convinced me that true male-type baldness in women is extremely rare and should be treated with great care.

Why does one testicle lie lower than the other?

If they were at the same level it would be like having a permanent conker game going on inside your boxers or jockeys. Think of that executive toy where you release one steel ball to drop on a line of four other balls – the one on the other end swings up and away with some force. Apply that thought to a man's testicles, and how tender they are, and you will gather why men with level-set testicles died out early in the process of human evolution.

Is a man's hand size really a sign of the length of his penis?

Who are you kidding? Who has done the research and how? What was the researcher's gender, and how did he/she go about the measurements? I'd love to read the paper, if there is one. My gut instinct here is that it isn't. (I have small hands.) There are men for whom huge hands are inversely related to the size of their penises. In other words, the bigger the hands the smaller the penis. I refer to bodybuilders who use steroids to build their muscles. As the chemistry of steroids is close to that of the male sex hormone testosterone, their testes get the message that no more work is needed from them. So they stop producing testosterone, and the penis responds in the normal way. It shrinks – sometimes almost out of sight. The bodybuilders don't seem to mind. I think most men – and their partners – may think differently.

How much exercise should we really do every day if we want to get fit?

You probably don't want to know this answer. Before we civilized ourselves, we were hunter-gatherers. The average male hunter walked and ran around 25 miles a day, the equivalent of a leisurely marathon. The female gatherer wasn't far behind at around 20. Once they had hunted and gathered their food, they ate it as fast as they could, then slept it off until they were hungry enough to go off and find some more food. So their lives alternated between satiation and starvation – and that's what our bodies are best suited for, even today.

But, I hear you say, we had a period of domestication of animals and farming after the hunter-gatherer period. Didn't our bodies change to suit that type of life? The answer to that is we haven't done it for long enough for the process of evolution to change us. Which is why, now that food is plentiful and we don't have to do so much exercise to catch or find it, we get fat and are prone to diabetes. Think of the poor Pima Indians.

Of course no one can be expected today to walk a marathon four or five times a week (three days a week our ancestors probably spent sleeping). But we still need to exercise enough to keep ourselves reasonably slim – and that, for most people, means an hour or so of brisk enough exertion to become breathless at least four times a week. Put your hand on your heart and say that you do that.

What was that about the Pima Indians?

They are a Native American tribe living in the arid desert area of the south-western United States. In around 1905 a study of them showed that they were still hunter-gatherers. They were all fit and slim, lived in relative poverty, but to an advanced old age. They didn't ask for much, and they didn't have much. Then someone discovered oil on their lands, and they made very astute deals with the United States government about its ownership. Virtually overnight they became rich. They bought cars and houses, ate very well, and lived a life of leisure and little manual work.

In one generation they became obese, almost every one of them – and disaster followed. They developed by far the highest rate of diabetes in the world, and they started dying of heart attacks and strokes in their thirties and forties. They nearly died out completely. Only with very good health education, and the realisation of the Pima themselves that they were in a terrible state, did they turn the corner. They are now eating healthily and are careful about their exercise levels, and thriving again. It's a huge success story that we in Britain could learn from, now that a third of our schoolchildren are defined as obese.

Is sweating when exercising a sign of being fit?

No, it's just a sign that you have exercised enough to put

your body heat up, and your body is trying to get it down again into the optimal range of around 37 degrees centigrade. You lose heat as the sweat evaporates from your skin surface: the spot from which the liquid disappears is cooled, and with this going on all over your body, the lower temperature is translated into your bloodstream. You only see a tiny proportion of your sweat: most of it evaporates before you can see it as a droplet on your skin. You will sweat just as much if you are unfit as if you are fit.

How do I know if I'm depressed?

That's an odd question. Do you have some doubts about low moods? Most people sense when they are depressed – they feel low, don't want to meet people, lose interest in things, and may start to do badly in their jobs. They wake up early in the mornings, and can't get to sleep again. They either lose their appetite or take refuge in overeating.

If you recognise two or more of these changes in yourself you are probably depressed and need help, preferably from your doctor. Without going into all these symptoms, however, there is an extremely simple but reliable exercise you can do yourself. Imagine a line drawn 10 centimetres long. At the 0 end of the line is deep unhappiness, where you see everything as black. At 10 you are blissfully happy, and see no clouds in your life. At 5 you are just so-so; 7 or 8 would be reasonably happy, 2 or 3 pretty miserable. Now put, without thinking much, your own number in that range.

If you score anything above 6 you are probably OK; 5 is beginning to be sad, verging towards depression; anything below 4 needs help; 2 or 1 needs urgent professional help. The modern treatment uses both drugs and a technique called cognitive behaviour therapy – but your doctor will introduce you to them.

Why, when I grow a beard, does it come out ginger?

I suppose you are more likely to notice ginger beards in men with hair of another colour, so they stand out. But only a minority of men in reality do have ginger beards. It may be because that part of their face doesn't produce melanin, but pheomelanin (of which more below). Why that should be is not easily explained.

In the past, if you had a ginger beard, you would certainly have wanted to shave it off. Prejudice against ginger has a long history. Right back to Judas Iscariot, in fact, who was said to be the only ginger-haired disciple. Naturally this has led to a fair amount of prejudice against red hair ever since – and it may still be there. In the witch-hunts of the 16th and 17th centuries many women were condemned to death simply because they were ginger. Here is the 17th-century French 'scholar' Jean-Baptiste Thiers in his book on the history of wigs:

> Redheads should wear wigs to hide the colour of their hair, of which everybody stands in horror because Judas was red-haired.

As for why men grow beards of any colour, there's the standard explanation that a beard proclaims a man's virility, and that, if you haven't proven yours by getting to the top in your job, you might as well do it in a simpler way by stopping shaving. Leave Bob Geldof out of it – he is hardly unsuccessful, and when was he last clean-shaven?

Still, it's worthy of note that in the world of politics almost all of the men who have become president or prime minister in the past hundred years have preferred glassily smooth chins. Maybe they didn't feel the need to proclaim their virility – they preferred the attraction of power instead. Fashions come and go, of course but today power is beardless.

Can your hair go white overnight, with shock?

Answering off the top of my head, it is very difficult to imagine how it could. When hair has become white, it's because the shaft of the hair has become hollow, and air is present throughout the shaft. The air gets in at the root, when the new hair is being produced, and after that nothing can change the composition of the hair. As hair grows only a little faster than nails, most of the hair on your head has been there for a few weeks. Only the hair nearest the scalp is new. So for hair suddenly to go white, it would need every hair suddenly to become hollow and full of air from base to tip overnight. When I was asked this question, I didn't know of any way in which this could happen. People can turn white fairly quickly when they reach their fifties, when the hair follicles, the structures in the skin that produce the hair, start to age. So it's normal for us to become white over several weeks – the time for air-containing hair to grow long enough to be the majority of the hairs on our head. But overnight? That, for me, was a different matter. Until I read the *British Medical Journal* of 6th May 2006.

In it, there are two photographs of a man whose hair turned white over a period of 36 hours – and a follow-up photograph six months later, of his hair back to its previous 'salt and pepper' appearance. How could this have happened? Dr Jessie Felton and Meg Price, skin specialists in Brighton, explained. He had a rare condition called alopecia areata, in which a change in his immune system caused very sudden hair loss, but only of the hairs which still contained their pigment. So all his pigmented hairs fell out over a day and a half, leaving just the white (hollow) hairs behind. Being left with only his white hairs, his hair had truly 'gone white' overnight (and had become much more sparse in the process). Alopecia areata can recover, and in his case the pigmented hairs eventually grew back, giving him his previous colour, and thick head of hair, again.

Whether a sudden shock can cause alopecia areata is still a matter of debate among doctors, but there are plenty of people with it who date their loss of hair to one – Duncan Goodhew, the Olympic swimmer, among them.

How can I improve my memory? I can't seem to remember names and numbers like I used to.

You can try going hungry for a few days. That's the message being put forward by researchers at Yale Medical School in the United States. When your stomach has been empty for a few hours, it starts to produce a substance called ghrelin, which finds its way into the bloodstream. Once it reaches the hypothalamus, a structure in the base of the brain, ghrelin triggers the chemical reactions that make us feel hungry.

That's simple enough to understand. If we have had an empty stomach for some time, we need to eat again fairly shortly, and the feeling of hunger is going to make us search for food.

So how does this affect memory? The Yale researchers found that ghrelin also 'latches on' to another area of the brain, the hippocampus, the centre for learning new things and memory. Mice injected with ghrelin greatly outperformed other mice in all sorts of tests for learning and memory – by as much as 40 per cent. The injected mice turned out to have a more complex brain structure than normal mice, with at least 30 per cent more connections between their brain cells – a strong indication that they had better brainpower and memory.

The researchers went further. They bred a strain of mice that couldn't produce ghrelin: these unfortunate animals underperformed in the memory and intelligence tests, but they improved dramatically when they were given the injections.

Human and mouse brains aren't hugely different in their basic chemistry, so the Yale team have already started giving some human volunteers injections of ghrelin to see if it has the same effect in them. If it works, drugs developed from it could make a big difference to illnesses like Alzheimer's disease and age-related memory loss. The team are also starving some human volunteers, to see if their stomachs' production of ghrelin improves their mental agility and memory.

One of the investigators, Tamas Horvath, suggests, not completely tongue-in-cheek, that if you are facing a hard day at work and need all your wits about you, you might try missing breakfast. The ghrelin response to even a few hours of starvation may make you sharper and more able to focus on your mental tasks.

And, though they run contrary to everything we have been told over the years about having a good breakfast, the results make sense. We all feel sleepy after a big meal, partly because we need to divert resources to our gut to deal with the process of digestion. That means less priority to other areas, like our muscles and brain. Our ancestors (those hunter-gatherers again) were designed, after a big meal in the wild, to hide away from predators and go to sleep. They simply shut down their memory and intellect by becoming unconscious. When they hadn't eaten for a while, and needed more nourishment, they needed all the brainpower they could muster to find their next prey. They had to switch on their intellect again to track their prey, their memory of where they found it last time, and the hunger to motivate them. Hunger, intellect and memory were three combined necessities to stay alive.

So eating only when you feel hungry, and never overdoing it so that you feel excessively sleepy afterwards, may be one way to stave off memory loss and deteriorating intelligence.

Can riding bicycles make men impotent?

It sure can. I hate to dissuade would-be Tour de France aspirants from their ambitions, but a fair proportion of professional long-distance cyclists are impotent, some permanently so, according to medical reports. The problem stems from the pressure that the hard, knife-like racing saddle puts on the perineum, the tissue between the base of the penis and the anus. The nerves that produce an erection pass through this area, and the hard saddle compresses them against the underlying bone. That can damage them permanently. So if you want to cycle, use a saddle that doesn't do this. There are new designs of divided saddle that take the pressure off the perineum: I'm amazed that they aren't more popular. It seems that winning prizes in the racing world can be more important to the top professionals than their sex lives. However, if you are thinking of riding a normal bike for pleasure, and have a comfortable saddle, you don't need to worry. You need many hours of riding on a really hard saddle several days a week for many months to ruin your manhood.

The Neurotic Mother

She's easy to spot. She's always running a little late for the party, and looking a bit rough around the edges – and when you get to talk to her (when she's finally off her mobile after checking on her brood for the fifth time) you realise that she thinks and breathes the bringing up of her children. She looks on every new medical scare story as if it affects her personally, so if Rocky Mountain Spotted Fever breaks out in some school camp in Arizona, she is sure her child has it. She is scared of allergies, viruses, cancer, autism, and her child going out to play. She joins every disease pressure group. Her husband or partner is long-suffering and silent, and, if he is with her, tends to hide in a corner, suffused with embarrassment, usually behind a large glass of gin.

My children hardly sleep at night. Is it true that this could stunt their growth?

In theory it could. We only produce growth hormone when we are asleep, so we grow mainly when we are asleep, and our growth slows down when we are awake. So if your children are really not getting enough sleep, their eventual adult height could be up to two inches less than their potential. However, they would have to lose a lot of sleep to make that much difference. Keep the video games and television out of the bedroom, and cultivate good bedtime habits for them. They are mainly common sense.

What is worse in a child: a very high temperature that lasts a relatively short time, or a lower fever that goes on for longer?

Interesting question. We have to go back to the days before antibiotics and fever-reducing drugs to find the answer. Before sulphonamides and penicillin, people expected children with infections to have high fevers. They watched until the temperature was at its highest, then hoped for it suddenly to fall. That high point was called the 'crisis' – Hippocrates used it in his descriptions of disease nearly three thousand years ago. The crisis was resolved in one of two ways – the child recovered or died. Which explains why the word has come into general use as a point of extreme stress. Crisis, in Hippocrates's terms, was followed by 'lysis' (recovery) or death.

As for the fever, it is caused by the body's effort to kill off the invading germs, on the principle that we can survive a higher temperature rise than they can. It may be a small window of safety – the bugs die off at, say, 40 degrees, and we can survive to 42. So if we throw a fever of 41, we win. We may not win, however, if we have to climb to 43 or higher – then we *and* the bugs (because they die if we do) are the losers.

As for a lower temperature that seems to drag on, that's a different matter. It is usually a sign of a continuing low-grade infection. Often in children (particularly girls) it's in the kidneys, so if your child is 'under the weather' or hot and sweaty, or headachy and shivery, with aches and pains in the limbs and back, and her temperature is 38 or above, you need to seek help. Your doctor will check ears, nose and throat, chest, kidneys and urine to rule out the common causes.

Not all fevers are caused by infection: there are other illnesses, mainly of the lymphatic system and bone marrow, in which people have high temperatures every few days or so. Your doctor will usually take blood tests to rule them out, too.

So what do we do for fevers? Today, we don't have to

wait and watch, like Hippocrates. We have antibiotics to deal with specific infections, and we have fever-lowering drugs, like the non-steroidal anti-inflammatory drugs ('NSAIDs' such as naproxen and indomethacin), to make people feel more comfortable and reduce the temperature. Aspirin is probably still the most effective for adults (we don't use it in children nowadays). For children with high fevers, keeping them cool with a fan is effective. Some children convulse when their temperature rises too high, so they need special care to avoid the 'crisis' stage.

Is it true that, if a young child gets burnt twice in the same place from the sun, then they are likely to get skin cancer?

No, it's not. But every time you do allow yourself to be sunburnt you raise your risk of developing a skin cancer. As the face and the back of the hands are the areas most exposed to the sun, they are the areas of skin most likely to develop cancer. The earlier you start burning yourself (as in childhood) the more likely you are to have a cancer. So children, particularly, should be protected by floppy hats, shirts and suncreams.

Once and for all: are dummies really bad for babies?

I have spent most of my years as a doctor condemning dummies as dirty things that would deform, and cause decay in, children's developing teeth and as a substitute for good maternal attention. So I would strongly argue against them having any benefit at all. I have come to appreciate, with time, that they might have their uses, particularly in keeping a yelling child quiet in the surgery. Nevertheless I have always thought the drawbacks outweighed the benefits – until a report in the *British Medical Journal* on 7th January 2006, which suggested that there were fewer cot deaths among children given dummies overnight than among non-dummy users.

The Californian group of Li De-Kun, Marian Willinger and their colleagues compared the dummy use of 185 infants who had died suddenly and 312 'control' living infants in the same area. There were fewer deaths among dummy users than among non-dummy users. The authors suggest that the dummies keep the babies on their backs and perhaps stop the babies choking while they sleep.

Should I now change the views of a lifetime? I'm not sure. The article provoked some stinging responses from doctors who interpreted the results in different ways, including the possibility (not calculated for) that some of the non-dummy users might have used dummies on other nights but, being ill on the night that they died, behaved unusually and did not accept their usual dummy. I'm still not recommending dummies to my patients.

How dangerous is it, really, to live under power lines?

A few years ago, when there was concern about leukaemia rates near nuclear power stations and secret army sites, a group of researchers looked at the reported rates of deaths from bone marrow diseases near several military structures. They showed conclusively that there were several areas close to massive military structures with high leukaemia counts. Unfortunately for the people wanting to take issue with the Ministry of Defence, many of them were castles built by the English to subdue the Welsh in the 12th century!

They were making the point that it was difficult to prove beyond doubt that clusters of cancers and leukaemias in any area were related to spills of radiation. As with magnetism, it is very difficult to connect power lines with any effect on human beings except that they cause a lot of anxiety. No one has yet proved conclusively that they do any harm.

Is it true that if you measure a child's height at their third birthday, their final height will be exactly double it?

You have the wrong birthday. It's actually the second birthday, not the third. Two-year-olds are taller than you think they are! A child who is three feet tall on his or her second birthday will be around six feet, give or take an inch, when an adult. That works for girls and boys. The height they are at any other age is much more difficult to correlate with adult height. For example, a girl who is very tall for her age at 10, but who has an early start to her periods, may end up smaller than girls who have a later start to their periods.

We put on most height at the start of puberty: it's called the growth spurt. The older girls and boys are when they start on their growth spurt, the more inches they gain during it. So a growth spurt starting at 14 is likely to put on several inches more than one starting at 11. As the mature sex hormones 'kick in' in girls, growth stops. Growth continues for a few years more in boys, which is the main reason that men are taller than women.

I always get a cold and cough after I've been on an

aeroplane flight. Is that a coincidence?

No, it's probably not. The inside of a pressurised aeroplane with 300 people on board is the perfect environment for the spread of respiratory viruses and even bacteria. The air is only partly filtered or replaced before it is returned to you. So one person sneezing in the cabin means that everyone has the pleasure of sharing his or her viruses within a few minutes. In any 300 people, several are likely to be harbouring cold viruses or worse in their throats. So if you haven't had a cold from that particular virus in the past (see the question on colds), you are going to get it in the next 48 hours. There's no escape.

A few years ago, a woman with open tuberculosis boarded a plane that landed in Britain. Two women seated several rows ahead of her developed the same strain of tuberculosis, with the same pattern of drug resistance, within a month of the flight. So we do take a risk (though very small in the case of tuberculosis) whenever we fly. It's one we are usually willing to take.

Why are some moles raised and some flat – is one type more risky than another?

'Moles' are more properly called pigmented naevi, and

most of us have quite a few of them (up to several hundred) if we look carefully enough. Some remain flat, like freckles, some are thicker than the surrounding skin and become raised above it. Most of us have the odd 'dermatofibroma' on our skin, perhaps on a leg or an arm. It is a small dome-shaped firm lump, which may or may not be pigmented (it's often pink), around two millimetres in diameter.

The vast majority of moles, whether flat or raised, are and remain harmless. Of course, the recent publicity about the sun and skin cancer has raised doubts about this statement, and people are constantly aware of the slightest change in their skin, especially if they have at some time had sunburn. So what are the changes that mean things have taken a turn for the worse?

Here are the latest guidelines from the American Cancer Society and Cancer Research UK on when to worry about a mole possibly becoming malignant and progressing to a 'melanoma': there are three major signs – changes in size, shape, and colour – and three minor signs – inflammation, crusting or bleeding; a feeling that it is different, or is painful, or itches; a diameter of seven millimetres or above.

All these changes can start in a flat or a raised naevus, so be alert to them. Usually a malignant melanoma has an irregular rather than a smooth edge, and the depth of the black, brown or blue colour varies across the surface, but if you have a mole with one or more of the 'majors' and one of the 'minors' above, you must see your doctor about it.

Above all, get to know your skin, so that you can detect a change in any part of it. How well do you really 'know the back of your hand'? Shut your eyes and try to picture it – the length of your fingers, the shape of the veins and tendons, the spots and hairs in your skin. Then open your eyes and see if you were anywhere close. You will be shocked by how far out you were.

So look at your skin once in a while and see if you can remember the pattern of moles. There are astronomers who look at the night sky and can, at a glance, pick out a new star, say a supernova, that wasn't there the previous night. It shouldn't be so difficult to do the same for your skin.

Are the white spots on my son's nails a sign of lack of calcium?

No, they're not. They are tiny air pockets lying between the skin under the nail and the undersurface of the nail. Your son probably knocked the nail against something, and didn't even notice when he did it. The tiny trauma has lifted the nail upwards, and left the white spot.

There are other nail problems, though, that you should heed. Developing a spoon-shaped depression in the nail, so that you could hold a droplet of water on it, is a sign of iron deficiency anaemia. That can have many causes, so if your nails are spoon-shaped, get a check-up. See your doctor, too, if you have small red flecks like tiny lines under the nails near the tips. These may be small 'emboli' (thromboses in small blood vessels – see page 76) from a heart problem. Ridges running lengthwise from cuticle to tip don't matter much. They are just the way the nails grow in some people. But if the ridges are at right angles to the growing direction of the nail, this may indicate times of ill health (the nails have stopped growing for a short time) and you should ask for a medical. If you have thickened finger ends, with nails that bulge out so that they look like small knobkerries (African clubs), these are called 'clubbing' fingers (not surprisingly) and are a sign of chronic lung or heart disease. If yours are like this, let your doctor see them.

I'm over 45 and haven't had a period for a year. Can I still get pregnant?

Most women go through the menopause in their late forties, but it isn't a precise date. You can still drop the odd egg into the womb at any time in the two years after your last period. Every doctor knows of women aged up to 50 who thought they were postmenopausal, and then found they were pregnant. It's rare for pregnancies to start normally (that is, not under the care of doctors who have deliberately treated women to ovulate) after 50, and the record for a natural pregnancy in British women stands at 53. My own oldest 'mum' had her 49th birthday on the day we delivered her nine-pound son. She was great about it, and says he has kept her young.

What's the best way to cope with travel sickness, particularly car sickness, in children?

The simple answer is to get them to pretend to drive the car. Drivers don't get car sick because they have to concentrate on the road ahead. If children can be persuaded to do that, then they won't get car sick, either. We have two mechanisms for knowing where we are relative to the space around us – our eyes and our balancing organs. In everyday life we use them together: their pathways to the brain work together so that it gets the same message from both of them. It's different when we are travelling in an enclosed vehicle. Our eyes may be concentrating on something inside the vehicle, while the balancing organs (fluid-filled semi-circular canals in the inner ear that act just like spirit levels) detect that we are moving on the road (or sea, or air, as the case may be). The brain gets confused – are we jiggling about in a car, or are we flowing along a road? The confusion leads to nausea and dizziness.

So the answer is simple – co-ordinate your eyes and spirit levels with the outside world, and not with anything inside the vehicle you are in. In a car that means looking at the road ahead. On a ship it means getting out on deck, if you can, and staring at the horizon. It's not so easy in a plane, but plane flights today are usually so steady that air-sickness is rare. If you are in a window seat, stare out at the clouds or the view below.

To get back to the children: in modern cars it's often difficult to see ahead from the back seat. So try to make sure that your children have good high safety seats that allow them to see out. Playing games like identifying cars or lorries on the way helps them to keep looking outwards, and books and video games should be banned.

Is asthma inherited? If so, is it more from the mother or father?

A disease may run in the family but not be inherited. In

Victorian times it was thought that tuberculosis was inherited because so many people in the same family had it. However, that turned out to be because people living in close conditions spread it easily from one to another. The tendency to have asthma (to possess the IgE system) is certainly inherited. Interestingly it is more likely to have been inherited from your father than your mother, something found out only recently. So look more into the father's than the mother's side for evidence of an asthma risk.

What is an inactive thyroid and what are the symptoms?

Your thyroid gland is wrapped around the front of your larynx, your voice box, and is the human body's equivalent of the accelerator in a car. It produces thyroid hormone (more accurately thyroxine, or even more accurately triiodothyronine), to the order of the pituitary gland, which hangs by a stalk from the base of your brain in a neat cavity in your skull. The pituitary gland secretes thyroid-stimulating hormone (TSH) into the blood-stream, where its rising levels are picked up by the thyroid gland. When the thyroid gland is stimulated, it then sends out the thyroid hormone into the blood – and that's where the fun starts. The more active your thyroid in its response to TSH, the faster your pulse, the faster you think, the more physically active you are, and the hungrier you are. An overactive thyroid leaves you hungry, physically active and mentally alert, with a fast heartbeat and as thin as a whippet. Even though you eat a lot, you burn off the extra calories so that you don't put on weight. In fact, one sign of an overactive thyroid is to lose weight while eating like a horse.

An inactive thyroid is the opposite. If TSH doesn't persuade it to come up with the goods, and it fails to produce thyroid hormone, then you slow down, mentally and physically. Your heart rate falls, you think more slowly, so much so that it has been confused with dementia, your features coarsen, your hair falls out, your skin thickens, and you put on weight even though you don't have a particularly good appetite. There are a host of other symptoms, but this isn't a medical textbook, and these are enough to be going on with.

Suffice to say that if your thyroid gland does pack up it is easy to replace the missing thyroid hormone by a simple pill containing it (usually in the form of thyroxine, though sometimes as triiodothyronine) once a day. The dose is determined by how you respond and you need to have blood levels taken of the hormones and of TSH every few months to make sure that you are still OK.

Why does the thyroid gland become inactive? Most

cases are due to an 'autoimmune disorder' in which the body's immune system thinks that the gland contains 'foreign material' that must be destroyed. The mistake is a costly one, leading to eventual destruction of the cells that produce thyroxine. Happily it isn't lethal, and modern treatment is extremely effective. Most people whose thyroid glands are diagnosed as underactive live normal lives once on treatment. If you want to know more about it, try my book on thyroid problems (Wellhouse).

How do you know when your menopause is starting?

That's another of those questions that need a whole book for an answer. The menopause usually covers a period of a few years from start to finish, and women all differ from each other in how it starts and how long it takes. The medical definition of the menopause is the time when the periods stop, but that's not easy to determine. Some women's periods stop suddenly, others become further and further apart until they eventually stop without the women knowing exactly when the last true period was. This can be difficult for contraception: I've known two women in their late forties who assumed, because they had had no periods for more than six and nine months respectively, that they were now past pregnancy. They weren't: fortunately both welcomed their new babies, as did their twentysomething brothers and sisters! Getting 'caught' at that age isn't uncommon – it happens to the most prestigious of women, among them the Queen and Cherie. There's a theory that women get a short surge of oestrogen just before their ovaries pack up for good, and that's the time they become pregnant.

For most women who have had regular periods, the menopause isn't much of a problem, despite the reams of magazine articles saying the opposite. Of course there are the hot flushes, the sweats, the change in sex drive (often it increases – certainly as often as it subsides) and the changes in mood. But, given an understanding of the process they are going through and the support of friends and partners, it isn't a bad time in life. It gives women the freedom not to have to worry about contraception, and often a new lease of married life.

Problems arise when the periods become heavier and more frequent, rather than slighter and less often. That's not normal and, if that's happening to you, you should see your doctor. It may mean fibroids in the wall of the womb or changes in the lining cells. Either case today is usually easily dealt with by a new technique to remove the womb lining by microwaves: hysterectomies for menopausal problems are almost a thing of the past, and thank goodness for that.

A rule of thumb for when to expect the menopause is that if you started your periods early, say at around 11 years old, you can expect them to go on longer, say until your late forties. If they started late, they may end a few years earlier. But this is such a rough guide that it can't really be forecast for each woman individually. Your mother's age at menopause might be a better guide, but only if you enjoy the same lifestyle as she did.

Should I really be paranoid about parabens?

Frankly, no. Parabens (technical name hydroxybenzoates) are just chemicals added to various skin preparations like ointments and creams to hold them together so that they spread easier. They are classified as 'excipients'. I've just looked them up in the *British National Formulary* (the doctor's 'bible' for prescribing) and they are present in a whole series of skin preparations, none of which in my experience has ever caused a problem with side effects. According to the medical establishment they are not carcinogens (they do not induce cancer in the standard tests). According to a 2006 edition of the *BNF*, 'they rarely cause problems. If a patch test indicates allergy to an excipient, then products containing the substance should be avoided.' I have never had to stop prescribing a cream or ointment containing parabens because of an allergic reaction.

So why are some people so worried about parabens? It has been claimed that antiperspirants containing them may cause breast cancer. The basis of the claim is that most women are right-handed and apply the antiperspirant to the left side with more force than they do to the right. Breast cancer, it is said, typically occurs in the left-hand upper segment. I have problems with this. First, it's not the force with which creams are applied that drives the constituents of creams, ointments or antiperspirants through the skin into the underlying tissues, where they must be if they are to cause a cancer. Penetration through the skin depends much more on the chemical properties of the application and the thickness of the skin at the point at which it is applied. There's no evidence that using your stronger hand will put more parabens into the underlying breast tissue than will your weaker hand.

Equally I know of no research that links a woman's handedness with cancer of the opposite (or the same, for that matter) side breast. There should have been a strong association if the claim was correct, as women have been using parabens in deodorants for many years now. There's a third point: it hasn't been shown that regular deodorant users have more breast cancers than non-users. Until I've seen these doubts answered with figures to prove the case I'll treat the parabens scare as just that. I'm willing to change my mind when I get more evidence. If you are still worried, then simply choose creams that don't contain them. But they have to have some additive to keep them smooth and easy to apply. Will this new additive have any better claim to safety than parabens? Or do we have to go through all these questions again, later, with this one?

Is it better to immunise your kids against everything with vaccines like MMR or is there an argument for encouraging an old-fashioned natural immune system? I got mumps and measles as a child.

More accurately, you *survived* mumps and measles as a child. Every doctor of my generation has seen children die from mumps and measles, and many more permanently disabled by them. We also saw people die from or be paralysed by polio, given permanently crippled chests by whooping coughs, and die young from the effects of diphtheria-induced heart disease. In Britain in the 1920s, tens of thousands of children died each year from infectious diseases. Thousands of babies were born blind, deaf and mentally disabled because their mothers had caught german measles (rubella) during their pregnancies. All these children depended on their 'old-fashioned natural immune systems' for their protection against disease. There is no argument to be made for it. None. None at all.

It seems that in just one generation we have forgotten all this crucial history. Because we don't see these diseases any more, we think we don't need the discomfort of a needle to be protected against them. We listen to the people (we have had them since the 18th century) who professionally oppose vaccination on warped evidence. We don't heed the rational voices of the people who have studied the figures, done the crucial research and are still watching people in the third world die from preventable diseases.

Here's an example of how twisted the anti-vaccination lobby can become. In 2005 religious leaders in sub-Saharan Africa ordered their flock to stop vaccinating their children against polio, which was on the verge of eradication. The result? An epidemic of paralytic polio that, carried by one or two pilgrims, spread from Africa to the Far East, affecting tens of thousands of children and adults. It is still there: in a part of the world from which vaccination had banished it years before.

You don't think that can happen here? The allegations (on very shaky claims by one doctor, not a specialist in immunity) that the MMR vaccination caused autism and bowel disease led to thousands of British and Irish mothers refusing the vaccine. Despite many studies refuting both claims and exposing the original research as wholly flawed, parents still refused to give the MMR vaccine. They didn't listen to the doctors who tried to explain that the whole basis of giving the three immunisations separately was a nonsense, without any immunological reasoning. You don't 'overwhelm the immune system' by giving three injections at a time, as some women fear. The immune system doesn't work like that. Each vaccine stimulates a separate set of immune reactions, which don't interfere with each other and don't put unnecessary strain on the immune system. Giving them separately is simply cruel, multiplying the number of injections by three. The child becomes terrified to see the health team because his or her life is dominated by injections. That makes the child-doctor relationship much more difficult later.

In Mexico, because they must inject children against many tropical infections, the health authorities give octovalent vaccines – eight vaccines in one injection. They don't see any greater reactions to the eight than we do to our three, and they have absolutely no opposition to this vital health protection.

The MMR fears resulted in measles outbreaks in Ireland, killing two children, and in Britain in the spring of 2006, killing another child and maiming many more. We saw measles in one of the practices with which I am involved for the first time in 20 years. They were very sick children. None had had an MMR. I would love the parents of the affected children to confront the doctor who started the anti-MMR campaign.

I don't know why we still have the vicious anti-vaccination lobby here. Alone in Europe we have forgotten our history. Our colleagues in Europe watch what happens here and sadly shake their heads. I've been doing a lot of head-shaking myself lately.

My son has had a bout of asthma twice after eating hamburgers and fizzy drinks at a well-known food chain. Could there be a link?

Yes, according to New Zealand doctors, who in 2005 reported a series of cases. It's still not clear whether it is the material in the burgers or in the drinks that causes the flare-up, but they describe it as 'significant' and advise people with asthma to be wary of fast foods.

Can I predict when my daughter is likely to start her periods from her weight and height?

Not from her height, but certainly from her weight: 95 per cent of all girls start to have periods when they reach between 46 and 48 kilograms in weight. It doesn't matter how tall they are. Tall girls who are slim start their periods later than small girls who are overweight. And as their eventual heights depend on making the menarche (the age at which periods start) as late as possible, this means that fatter girls will not be as tall as they might have been. It's another good reason for making sure that primary school children do not become overweight. Or develop anorexia nervosa.

Why bring in anorexia?

It's thought that one underlying reason for girls becoming anorexic is that subconsciously they fear becoming adult women. They want to postpone their periods for as long as possible.

So they keep their weight low enough – well under 47 kilograms – and remain childlike, without periods. I don't know if this is wholly accepted as one of the reasons for anorexia, but it is true that anorexic girls and women stop menstruating. The same used to be the case for those undersized girl athletes and gymnasts who trained so hard that they stayed tiny. Some of them found their ability to have children later was permanently damaged.

Why do I tend to moult in the winter and not in the summer?

Probably that's just your natural annual cycle of hair growth – our hair goes through phases of growth and resting, and yours happens to coincide with these seasons. Almost certainly it's nothing to worry about. One small point – maybe your thyroid gland is varying in activity, so that it is underactive in the wintertime. That would explain the fallout. You could always get it checked with a simple blood test. See the answer to the thyroid question. Trichologists often suggest to women losing their hair that they take iron tablets on the grounds that they are often a little anaemic (because of heavy periods), and that this causes hair loss. I'm not sure there is good medical evidence for this, but I know women who have been pleased with the result.

How bad are X-rays for you? I won't let the dentist X-ray my children because of the danger. Am I correct?

No. Modern dental X-rays deliver a tiny dose of radiation to a very focused area of your jaw. You are probably exposed to more radiation in your everyday life, perhaps from the granite rocks around you (in some areas they have a relatively high radium content) or from other radiation sources. The risk from the odd dental X-ray to you or your children is vanishingly small. You will see that modern dentists don't even put on lead aprons any more because the machines they use don't expose them to any excess that might harm them – and they are much more exposed to X-rays than you ever will be. Of course this doesn't mean people should be complacent about X-rays. They are innately dangerous, and if you are asked to have one, or a series of them, say, in hospital, do ask about the risk.

Can mobile phones really cause brain tumours?

At last we have the definitive answer to this scare – and it's no. Interviews with 966 British patients with gliomas, the commonest form of brain tumour, and the one that was suggested to be linked with mobile phone use, have shown that they didn't use a phone more often, or for longer, than 1,716 similar people, chosen randomly from family doctors' lists, who had no brain problems. Regular phone users had the same risk of a brain tumour as people who never or only occasionally used one. So we can put that scare firmly to rest, at least for a year or two. We haven't had mobile phones for long enough to rule out tumours arising after many years of use – but they seem increasingly unlikely.

OK, so they don't cause tumours, but can they cause worse headaches in people sensitive to them?

That's been studied, too. It's been claimed that some people are 'sensitive' to mobile phone signals, which can give them headaches or make their usual headaches much worse. So doctors from King's College Institute of Psychiatry devised an ingenious trial, exposing 60 'sensitive' people and 60 people ('controls') who didn't have such symptoms, to three conditions: – the usual mobile phone signal; a non-pulsing signal (it was believed that the pulse quality of the signal was the source of the headaches); and a 'sham' condition in which there was no actual electronic signal. Their subsequent headaches were then 'marked' for severity. The 'sensitives' developed headaches to all three conditions, and the non-sensitives reported few or no headaches at all. The 'sham' signal produced severe symptoms in some of the 'sensitive' test subjects, suggesting that they had underlying psychological, rather than physical, causes. Each of the three conditions provoked headache equally in the sensitive group, and had no effect in the others. So, whatever was causing the headaches in the sensitive subjects, it wasn't their mobile phones.

What are my chances of dying from a blood clot when I fly to New Zealand?

Pretty small really, especially if you fly Air New Zealand. They've got ample leg-room in economy (I have personal experience). But let me explain what it's all about, first. A thrombosis is a clot of blood that forms in your veins when the flow through them stagnates. Sitting for long hours with your legs bent and the front of the seat jammed into the backs of your knees can block the flow of blood upwards from your calves to your thighs. The bend in your hips, too, can cause the flow to become sluggish in the thigh veins. So the conditions are ripe for clots to form in the calves or the thighs, not just in aeroplanes, but in long distance buses, too. As long as the clot stays in the vein in which it is formed, it doesn't do much harm – it may cause a bit of pain and swelling in the calf or thigh, but eventually it disappears as the blood flow recovers.

The problem comes when a piece of the original clot in the leg breaks off and is swept upwards, through the heart, to the lungs, where it sticks and blocks the circulation in them. This is called an embolism, which makes you breathless and, if it is large enough, can kill you.

You would think, then, that thousands of air passengers would develop thromboses and embolisms every year. They don't. Emboli occur naturally in around one in 1,000 people every year in Britain, regardless of whether they fly or not. This is a relatively small medical risk. Among people who fly regularly for over 10 hours at a time, the risk remains very small, and difficult to assess for each individual.

The way we identify a thrombosis is to use a 'Doppler' ultrasound machine – it's simple and isn't invasive. One research team using Doppler found not a single thrombosis among 899 passengers flying for more than 12 hours. In another study, of 878 passengers who had travelled by air for 39 hours (I can't imagine where they had been), nine had signs of a thrombosis, of whom four had had an embolus. That's just 1 per cent, and of the nine, eight turned out to have been at extra risk (because of medical conditions) of a thrombosis before they flew.

It seems, then, that if you don't possess any of these medical 'risk factors', and are normally healthy, your risk of a life-threatening embolus on a long plane journey is extremely low. Still, it's best to know whether you are among the 'at risk' passengers. So here's your checklist. You are at extra risk of a thrombosis and embolus if you:

- smoke (any at all per day)
- have had recent major surgery
- have cancer
- are pregnant
- are taking the contraceptive pill or hormone replacement therapy (HRT)
- have varicose veins
- have had previous thromboses and emboli.

How do you lower your risk? Put on compression stockings (they should give 15 to 30 mmHg pressure at the ankle) before the flight. You can buy them at the airport or a pharmacy. Drink plenty of water (not alcohol, which dehydrates you further and promotes thrombosis) and move about during the flight. Even when seated, stretch your legs and move them about several times an hour. Lie as flat as you can, with legs stretched out, when you try to sleep.

If you know you are at very high risk then your doctor may advise an injection of low-molecular-weight heparin just before the flight. This will prevent a clot – but its side effects restrict it to people for whom a long flight makes a thrombosis almost inevitable.

So don't worry, but do see your doctor if you have a doubt about your fitness to fly.

Is it bad for your health to be on the contraceptive pill for a long time?

Wow. What a question. I've written a 35,000-word book on the subject, and you are asking me to condense it into one or two paragraphs. The answer, as in so many medical subjects, is 'It depends'. It depends on which pill you are taking (there are several types with different strengths and types of hormone), your lifestyle (whether you smoke, are obese, have high blood pressure, are at risk of a thrombosis), your family history (did a close relative have breast cancer?) and your own medical history (what illnesses have you had in the past?).

But let's assume that you are at no special risk, are relatively healthy, you don't smoke, are under 35, and are taking the low-dose combined pill (oestrogen and progestogen). In the first year of taking it you have a small extra risk of a clot (thrombosis) in a vein that could break up and end up in the lungs (an embolus). The numbers are tiny – five cases for every 100,000 women a year. That compares with a risk of 60 cases per 100,000 pregnant women a year, so it could be looked on as a saving if you were previously relying on, say, condoms or the rhythm method for your contraception (they aren't nearly as effective).

The risks are slightly higher on the so-called second and third generation pills (your doctor will tell you which pill belongs in which category) but they remain much lower than the risks with pregnancy. After a year of taking the pill, the risk of a thrombosis lessens.

However, it increases fairly sharply if you are overweight, you smoke and are over 35. If you smoke and are over 35 then the risk becomes so high that you have to stop one or the other. Your doctor will not prescribe the pill if you continue to smoke, as this would be irresponsible. You have to make the choice yourself.

A lot has been made about the increased risk of breast cancer for those on the pill. In fact, the risk is very small, amounting to a very few extra cases in 10,000 women taking it. And the extra cases only appear to occur in women in the first 10 years of taking it – so that women who have been on the pill for longer than that time have the same risk as women who have never taken it.

There are two points about the extra cases. They are almost always 'early' cases – that is, they are confined to the breast and eminently curable, so that they don't cause an excess death rate. This suggests that the women would have got the cancers anyway, but that they are diagnosed earlier when they are taking the pill – possibly because they are much more aware of breast problems and examine themselves more thoroughly than other women.

The second point is that the increased numbers of breast cancers associated with being on the pill are offset by reduced numbers of cases of ovarian cancer (which is, case for case, more lethal than breast cancer) and of uterine cancer. The pill appears actively to prevent womb and ovarian cancer. And, in very large studies, one unexpected but consistent result has been that women who have taken the pill for years have a much lower rate of rheumatoid arthritis. The hormones in the pills may help in some way to protect joints from the disease.

Then there is high blood pressure. In some women (again only a few) the blood pressure begins to rise when they go on the pill. If the rise were to continue, then they would be at higher than normal risk of a heart attack or stroke. However, it only rises slowly over time, so that a small rise can be recognised early and reversed. As with thrombosis, if the pressure is going to rise it usually happens in the first few months, but it *can* start to rise later, so you will need a twice-yearly blood pressure check all the time you are on the pill.

So is it bad for your health to be on the pill? Not if you know about the risks and take action when it's necessary. Huge studies of populations who have and haven't taken the pill suggest that the pill-takers live marginally longer. So it can't be too bad for you.

If my mother found giving birth easy, will I be the same?

I can understand your anxiety, but I can't give complete reassurance. If you have inherited the same pelvic shape as your mum, you are of the same general fitness as your mum was, and you have your first baby at around the same age as your mum did, then your labour is more likely than not to be similar to hers. But if you are five or more years older than she was at the time she had her first, then it's likely to be longer and a bit more exhausting. The longer you delay your first child, especially after your late twenties, the longer and more difficult your labour is likely to be. On the plus side, we are better able to alleviate the pains and difficulties of labour than in your mum's time, and women like yourself may well be fitter and have more effective antenatal care than she did, and that may make up for your age difference. Frankly, it's better, physically, for you to start a family in your early twenties, but plenty of women do well even when they give birth for the first time in their forties.

If my child is going to end up doing one or the other, which is best – drink or drugs?

What a question. Do you want to leave your child in the frying pan or throw him or her directly into the fire? Presuming that the frying pan is slower to kill than the fire, then alcohol is the first and drugs the second. Although it depends on what your child does while drinking. In my lifetime as a GP I've seen many more young lives wrecked by alcohol than by drugs, but that's only because in our area of Scotland, alcohol was far more easily available. Early deaths from booze are usually related to traffic accidents, with the occasional lethal overdose from small children drinking the contents of their parents' cocktail cabinet while they were out (and the babysitter was presumably asleep). Only in the past few years have we seen the results of teenage booze sessions (a relatively new phenomenon in our society) being translated into liver failure, with desperately ill young adults needing transplants (usually dying before one becomes available). So I wouldn't choose excess drinking as a pastime for any child.

But I would be even more concerned about drugs. We have read all the tragic stories about the sudden deaths from Ecstasy, and we brush them aside because they won't happen to our nicely brought up children. We don't believe that cannabis (marijuana, joints, hash, bhang or any of its fashionable and cosy word equivalents) really does any harm – and in any case, isn't it going to be used as a medicine for MS sufferers? That surely means it's really OK, doesn't it? And the glitterati all use cocaine, don't they? It doesn't seem to harm them, does it?

Here's what I think. It isn't fashionable, but it's taken

from my experience as a working GP in the first decade of the 21st century. Our area of rural Scotland has been totally transformed by the illegal drugs epidemic since the 1980s. We now have hundreds of heroin addicts – who all started on so-called 'soft' drugs, the initial one being almost always tobacco. We have teenagers damaged by 'E' and who are permanently under the supervision of the local psychiatric services purely because they tried cannabis. Many of these drug abusers have been in jail because they stole or worse to keep up their habits. They are all physical and mental wrecks with hardly any prospects of a reasonable quality of life. Many will die young in poverty and alone. When they come to us for help, we try our best, but with little hope, because we know the grip their drugs have on them, and the pressures their peers and their pushers exert upon them. They have lost any feeling for anything but how and where they can get their next fix.

What would I choose between drugs and alcohol? If I had to do so, then on balance I would prefer the child to take alcohol, because it is easier to try to control, and it is more openly available legally. (Don't take that as meaning I would like drugs to be legalized – I wouldn't.) People with alcohol problems are more likely to admit them, and to seek help for them. Drug abusers, in my experience, are much more likely not to see the problems the habit is causing, and very much less likely either to seek help or to

84

take it when offered. Frankly, I despair when I have to be involved with their care – and I know many other doctors who feel the same. I don't get quite that feeling of despair and hopelessness when I am dealing with an alcoholic.

Is it true that if you have been trying to start a family for more than a year, you are more likely to have a boy than a girl?

If you are Dutch, it appears so. I don't know whether it applies to all couples. Dutch doctors followed up 5,283 women who gave birth between 2001 and 2003. The couples who had taken more than a year to become pregnant (despite trying their hardest, so to speak) had more boys than would have been expected by chance. In any community, slightly more boys than girls are born. Usually the rate is 51 per cent boys and 49 per cent girls. That was the case for the couples who had succeeded in becoming pregnant within a year of trying to conceive. But for the women who had more than a year to wait, the boy:girl ratio was 57:43. This is big enough to be remarkable, but obviously not big enough to predict with any certainty that any individual who has had to wait will have a boy.

Why the difference? In some relatively infertile women,

the main barrier to conception is thicker than usual mucus in the cervix and womb. The Dutch doctors propose that male sperm (carrying the Y chromosome), being lighter and swimming faster than the female sperm (bearing the heavier X chromosome) can swim through this thicker mucus more easily – and therefore have a better chance of reaching the waiting egg. If this answer seems a bit 'far out', don't write to me about it – ask the obstetrics team in Maastricht.

Is it good for my children's brain development to expose them to more than one language at an early age?

That was a big bone of contention in Scotland in the early 20th century, when Gaelic, the native language of the Highlands, nearly died out because parents were told not to use it at home as it would hold back their children's education in English. Teachers punished any child heard using it in the classroom. Now we know better. The earlier you introduce a child to a second language, the more skills in language (and for ease of learning a third and fourth language later) they attain. It turned out that children proficient in both Gaelic and English found learning a third language like French easier than their schoolmates.

Gaelic is now enjoying a resurgence in Scotland. There's evidence, too, that a second language improves reasoning abilities, and perhaps even intellect. But it's not just exposing children to languages early that helps. Those who are trained in music develop extra skills in sorting out sounds – not just the musical notes, but words as well. So a child who is taught to appreciate and play music is more likely than most to be especially proficient in learning new languages.

How long should we wait between pregnancies? What's best for mum – and for the babies?

If you want to know about making labour as easy as possible, you have plenty of leeway. Best time for avoiding a difficult labour is between 18 months and five years after the previous one. Before 18 months, there's a little more bleeding: after five years, labour tends to be longer and more exhausting. Yet these are tendencies and not hard and fast rules. If you are thinking of how the children are going to get on together, then every two years is about right. They have little in common during their childhoods if they are spaced out beyond, say, every four years, and they may be too close as rivals if they come along every year. But again, these are tendencies – much depends on how the parents cope. Of course if you are thinking of having a rugby team, then the older children tend to look after the younger ones. This isn't so far-fetched: in the early years of the 20th century it was common to have between nine and 12 children, and they didn't get along too badly on the whole. In one of the happiest (and poorest, financially) families I had the privilege of looking after, the mother had had 19 children. They had three council houses knocked together into one. Everyone looked after everyone else, and Mum was slim and delightful in her mid-forties.

Paranoid Party Animal

Paranoid Party Animals enjoy life to the max. This includes copious amounts of wine (though they know that they exceed the government's weekly recommendation), far too many cigarettes (though they are definitely giving up next new year) and the odd recreational drug ('odd' being used rather loosely here).

The unfortunate downside to the PPA's otherwise hedonistic existence is 'dawn paranoia' – that terrified 3.30am moment, usually brought on by dehydration and a hammering head. Awake and hung-over, they are racked with anxieties about their lifestyle and health, and resolve to change IMMEDIATELY. Off they trot for a detox smoothie and a bag of pumpkin seeds . . . only to find that it's soon 7pm again, and an ice-cold glass of something rather delicious is in front of them and all their resolve is evaporating into the ether (or a haze of cigarette smoke).

I usually spot PPAs a mile off – and they are a complete lost cause. Afraid to tell their own GP the truth, lest he insist on an instant lifestyle change, they seek me out at parties, in desperate need of reassurance that the government warnings for some reason won't apply to them. I never spend too much energy on my replies as I know that, by the morning, they won't remember having talked to me anyway.

Will smoking dope make me thick?

Yes, despite what potheads claim. If you want to retain your memory and intellect, don't smoke or take marijuana in any form. Doctors in Greece have compared the mental abilities of 20 people who had smoked dope four times a week for 15 years with 20 who had used it for less than seven years, and 24 never-smokers. They were all given 15 words to memorise, then asked to repeat them later. The average score for the long-term pot-smokers was seven, for the shorter-term smokers it was nine, and for the never-users it was 12. This is a big difference, showing a lot of brain loss due directly to the drug. It is only the latest in many studies showing that repeated 'soft' drug abuse damages the brain. It isn't surprising that it does, because the main active ingredient of marijuana, tetrahydro-cannabinol, or THC, is highly fat-soluble. As our brain is the organ in our body with the highest concentration of fat, THC makes a beeline for it, and stays there for weeks. If you are a regular cannabis user your brain is never free of it – and that can make for long-term disaster, including psychosis (such as schizophrenia and paranoia), depression and dementia. Serious stuff.

So if you are a 'recreational' pot-smoker, please remember (before you forget) that your brain is your most precious asset. Damaging it permanently with pot just isn't worth it.

Why do I want to eat a horse on a hangover?

That's an interesting one. Most people can't look food in the face when they are hung-over – it just makes them feel sick. I don't know for sure the answer to this question, but I can suggest a possible one. Whether we are hungry or not depends on the levels of a substance called leptin in our blood. Leptin is released by fat cells into the circulation after we have started to eat a substantial meal. When it reaches the brain, it attaches to nerve cells in the 'hunger centre' deep in the brain. This effectively switches off our feeling of hunger, and we stop eating.

Brilliant, you are thinking. Why don't we use leptin to lose weight? Take a dose of it, switch off our hunger mechanisms, and slice off the pounds. Sadly, it doesn't work that way with obese people. They produce a lot of leptin naturally, but they also produce a protein called CRP in fairly large quantities – and this 'mops up' the circulating leptin before it has a chance to bind to the hunger cells. So they don't switch off their hunger. The more leptin we give to an obese person, the more CRP they produce, so that giving leptin will never be the answer for them. Now just maybe, when you (and not the other people who don't feel ravenous after a hangover) drink alcohol, it makes you produce extra CRP, which keeps you hungry. If that's so, I would avoid getting hungover, because rising CRP may mean early liver damage or inflammation of the liver, and that could be a prelude for worse to come.

Why do I get the munchies when I smoke dope?

Same answer as above, except for alcohol read dope. Same message, too. If dope is making you feel hungry, then your liver may be objecting. Maybe it's time you reviewed your lifestyle and whether or not you want a reasonably long life. There's a good reason for it to be called 'dope'.

What's the best way to get rid of a hangover?

If you're expecting one, then drink plenty of water now, and stop the booze for the night. The hangover is a combination of dehydration and dropping alcohol levels in the brain. The first is glaringly obvious and well known, but the second has subtler, sometimes even alarming, effects. If you can hydrate yourself, and limit the brain alcohol level by stopping your drinks now, you may just be OK.

The headache part of a hangover results from the dehydration – the brain shrinks a little with the dehydration, and that stretches the membranes around it. The pain nerve endings are in these membranes, and that gives you the headache. Keep the brain well watered and less oiled, and you could avoid it. The nausea is caused by the alcohol poisoning of the stomach and gut. You avoid that only by not drinking enough to reach poison levels. This is different for each individual but, as a general rule, four or five standard drinks over a few hours are enough to produce considerable ill-ease in most women, and a little more than that will do the same for most men. If you have drunk enough to be plastered, it takes a long time for your brain to recover.

Also, it is good to remember that overnight you lose only about 10 per cent of the alcohol each hour, so you may still be well over the limit for driving legally when you waken the next morning. At that point your brain is heavily sedated and still dehydrated, and it is fairly slow getting back to normal. Your reactions won't be right until maybe the early afternoon.

Hair of the dog as a remedy works in the short term, as a small amount of alcohol keeps the brain's alcohol levels higher, but it is probably also the way forward to alcoholism. Once you start to take alcohol in the mornings to treat alcohol withdrawal, you are well on the way to never being without it.

With apocryphal cures, such as Prairie Oysters or spicy Bloody Marys, remember that your stomach lining has had a battering. Alcohol has a direct effect on the stomach and it can take a day or two for the lining cells to recover from the insult. Anything that needs digesting – like raw eggs and dairy products – will just prolong this damage.

Why do I sometimes have a killer hangover and other times not, even when it seems I have drunk the same amount?

A lot depends on whether you have allowed yourself to be

dehydrated while doing the drinking the previous night. Headaches after drinking are as much about disturbing the normal balance of water and electrolytes (sodium, potassium, chloride, bicarbonate and other 'charged' molecules in your bloodstream, brain and other tissues) as about the level of alcohol. Hangovers sometimes depend, too, on the level of the 'higher' alcohols in what you have been drinking. In some drinks, mainly distilled spirits, it isn't only simple ethyl alcohol that blasts your suffering brain – there are many more complex molecules in the drink as well, and they can act as brain poisons. They are not too far from drinking petrol – which itself is only a 'higher' alcohol.

For example, for some completely unfathomable reason, absinthe has become popular as a drink among young people today. It was banned for years because it was known to be poisonous and even lethal in doses not much higher than a standard drink of it. We have seen terrible reactions to it in practice, with hangovers lasting days, and even one death.

So it isn't just the amount you drink, but what you drink, too. And whether someone has 'spiked' your drink. The morning after, do you really know what you drank the previous night? If you drank enough to have a killer hangover, I bet you don't.

It also depends on how fast you drank the alcohol: drinking a lot in a relatively short time raises your brain alcohol levels much higher than drinking slower, over several hours. Your headache comes when you start to become conscious again, and your brain becomes sensitive to the poison you have put into it. I have to say I'm not over-sympathetic to the questioner. The obvious answer is always to be in control of the amount you drink, so that you don't have a hangover. But I realise I'm just a fuddy-duddy grumpy old man who was never young himself.

Which is more likely to spread infection – kissing or shaking hands?

Until two or three years ago I'd have said kissing, but not now. Shaking hands can be bad news. Take winter vomiting virus, for example. It spreads rapidly among communities and in hospitals, causing diarrhoea and vomiting for two days; then the numbers of cases die away, so that it seems to have disappeared completely. It's only recently that the researchers have discovered what causes it, and how it is spread – and they have had a few surprises on the way.

We used to assume that most infections that lead to vomiting and diarrhoea are caught from food. If the stomach and gut are upset, it is natural that we should seek the cause in what has gone into them. Yet years of examining kitchens and foodstuffs dispensed in infected hospitals, for example, did not identify the cause.

Then cruise lines reported outbreaks of a very similar illness. Their kitchens were spotless, and the researchers agreed, as with the hospital outbreaks, that the cause could not have been due to bad hygiene among the staff. Nor did the season matter. Although the illness was called winter vomiting disease, it happened at any time of the year. Cruise ships stay away from wintertime, yet there have been dozens of outbreaks on them. Some cruises were even abandoned because so many passengers and crew were affected.

The breakthrough came when a virus, first called Norwalk, then norovirus, was found in the sample material from its victims. It wasn't found in the kitchens or in the food, but on the hands of people with the illness, as well as in their diarrhoea. Often it wasn't found in the saliva. It became clear that the virus spread from hand to hand. Someone incubating the virus could leave it on a door handle or a banister, or on cutlery, and that would be enough to infect the next person.

This was a revelation, because it was the general opinion of specialists that viruses, unlike bacteria, which are very different types of germ, could last only a short time outside the body, and would certainly die very quickly when lying on the skin of the hands – which has its own protective mechanisms for dealing with germs. It hadn't been thought possible that a handshake or a door handle could transmit a viral infection.

So cruise lines sent letters to every potential passenger saying that they must not board their ships if they had diarrhoea and sickness. They installed alcohol-based hand-washing systems at the entrance of their dining rooms. They offered free medical care if any passenger developed sickness and diarrhoea while on board, provided that they immediately informed the ship's doctor. Cruise-ship outbreaks of norovirus have lessened since these precautions began, although in the summer of 2006 there have been three in ships sailing out of Britain.

Hospitals are doing the same. But where cruise ships have a captive population that can be controlled, hospitals don't have that luxury. They have loads of visitors, and it has to be said that the initial norovirus infection that starts off hospital outbreaks is almost always brought in by patients' visitors. The lesson is not to visit a friend in hospital if you have recently been ill yourself or have recently been in the company of someone who has been ill. And wash your hands thoroughly before you get to the ward.

This knowledge isn't entirely new. It's said that Queen Victoria once sacked the royal doctor because he washed his hands only after examining her, and not beforehand. She was absolutely right to do so! Goodness knows where a Victorian doctor might have put his hands before he came to see the Queen. Especially if, as some still suspect, he was Jack the Ripper.

What about glandular fever – famous for being the 'kissing infection' in teenagers? Certainly the virus that causes it (it has the exotic name of Epstein-Barr) does pass from lip to lip. The other almost universal infection probably transferred by kissing is the cold-sore virus (herpes labialis). The oddest aspect of mouth infections, though, is our complete lack of knowledge about what causes mouth ulcers (aphthous ulcers). Almost everyone has had at some time these painful little white spots on the inside of the mouth, on the tongue or on the inside of the lips or cheeks, yet we don't know what, if anything, transmits them, or even if they are an infection. No one has ever found a virus or other germ to be responsible for them. The most effective treatment is to put a small tablet of cortisone on them. This removes the pain almost instantaneously, suggesting that the area is inflamed (cortisone is the ultimate anti-inflammatory drug), though we don't know what stimulates the inflammation in the first place.

I just drink wine: I don't touch spirits. Surely that will protect my liver?

Not necessarily. It depends entirely on how much alcohol

you drink. It doesn't really matter which type of booze you prefer. It's entirely about how much alcohol you take in each day, not how it's packaged.

How about milk thistle for your liver? Will this really help?

What do you expect milk thistle to do for your liver? A normal healthy liver doesn't need any form of medication, whether it is herbal or orthodox. It just gets on with its myriad jobs as usual. There isn't a magic ingredient in any medicine that can improve its performance as long as you are eating a varied diet and not abusing it with, say alcohol or, indeed, some of the herbal medicines that we have seen over the years which damage it. I remember the outbreak of liver disease among Afro-Caribbean children in Birmingham in the 1960s and 1970s because their mothers gave them 'bush teas' in the tragically mistaken belief that they were good for them. Then, a few years ago, several adults in Belgium suffered liver and kidney failure because of herbs imported from China.

I have to say that the Chinese community here is trying to put that right. What appears to have happened in Belgium, according to my favourite informant, is that the global popularity of Chinese herbs caused them to be over-harvested, and therefore scarce. Crooks got into the business of marketing and selling them, using substitute herbs that turned out to be poisonous. As a consequence of the Belgian cases, Kew Gardens has set up a special research centre, funded by the Chinese community in the UK, to analyse imports.

No, I wouldn't advise milk thistle for the liver or for any other organ. Health isn't like that. You are either eating healthily and living a healthy lifestyle, in which case you don't need any herbal or other supplement to improve your health, or you are sick. If you are the latter, isn't it wiser to trust the medical profession who know about organs and their problems? Just think of an 'alternative' aircraft engineer – would you like to fly in a plane designed by one of them?

When do we really need to see the doctor for a cough?

If you are a non-smoker, any cough that goes on for more than two to three weeks needs investigation. Your doctor will want to look at your throat and nose, and listen to your chest and take things further from there. If you are a smoker, you will have a cough anyway. Stopping smoking should stop the cough within a month. If it doesn't, then see your doctor. You will need to have your lung damage assessed. If you have a permanent cough and continue to smoke, you would be better talking to your lawyer about your will than to your doctor.

Can drinking wine be healthy?

It all depends on how much you drink. The evidence in favour is all down to Jean-Marc Orgogozo, a professor at Bordeaux University, who first told the world that alcohol was good for us. He had set out to prove once and for all how much harm red wine did to the population served by his hospitals. He had the perfect subjects all around him – a large number of people who had drunk wine every day from childhood, and a fair proportion who did not drink it at all. So he set up a huge study of almost everyone in his region, noted their drinking habits, then followed them for the next quarter-century. Every death certificate came under his department's scrutiny.

The result astonished him – and every other physician who heard him read his paper. The people who drank a moderate amount of red wine lived longer than those who had been teetotal. Not just a little longer, but several years longer. Long enough for the difference to be very significant. The odds that his results were produced by chance were more than 20 to one against. The red wine drinkers had far fewer heart attacks and strokes, and if they didn't overdo their habit, if they stuck to two or three glasses a day, they didn't even have a higher rate of liver disease. The trouble with this happy finding is that the average amount of red wine drunk by each partygoer in one night is often as much as Jean-Marc's 'moderate drinkers' swallow in a week.

The other side of Jean-Marc's conclusions should frighten, not reassure us. Ultimately, whether drinking wine can be healthy depends on what part of the J-curve you are on, a curve that relates the amount you drink with your risk of dying earlier than you would expect. It looks like the capital letter J. There's a little upward curve to the left, where the teetotallers are, and a much bigger and steeper curve upwards to the right, where the people are who drink more than two glasses of wine, or its equivalent, a day. The bottom of the curve – the people who live the longest – is a very precise point. It includes those who drink one or two glasses a day. The more you drink above that, the further to the right and the higher on the J you are. The higher you are, the shorter your life.

Three glasses today are bigger, by the way, than they were when Jean-Marc wrote about them in the 1980s. Wine glasses have ballooned in size. They used to contain 125ml wine. Now most take 250ml with ease. That is a third of a bottle of wine, or two standard glasses. Three glasses that size are six to eight units, depending on the strength of the wine, or enough alcohol for three whole days. If you are drinking three glasses of wine several times a week, you have climbed halfway up the big arm of the J.

I have read lots about the 'good things' in red wine, like lycopenes – the ones we also get in tea, tomatoes, apples and red onions? Don't they protect us?

It's true that all these foods contain substances that will help protect against a heart attack or stroke, but you aren't going to benefit if you, as a female, drink more than two small glasses of wine a day. Your liver can't cope with more than that load of alcohol. It's all very well protecting yourself against a heart attack, only to die earlier from liver cirrhosis. In any case, the real protection from drinking wine is the alcohol that's in it, not the other chemicals.

Is it true that drinking vodka with cheese fondue can kill you?

Why would you want to drink vodka with a cheese fondue? In fact why do you want to eat a cheese fondue in the first place? It's such a messy, unsatisfying meal. I don't know of any scientific reason why you can't drink vodka with one. Unless you drink so much vodka that you can't swallow easily and the melted cheese sticks in your throat, so that you choke to death. Trying to get sticky cheese out of the throat of a choking, panicking person isn't easy. The Heimlich manoeuvre won't work very well if the cheese is plastered around the tonsils and epiglottis, and glued down on to the opening of the larynx, and you have only seconds to stop asphyxiation. However, I've never had any occasion to do such a thing, so I don't suppose it is very common, and I can't find any direct reference to it in the medical literature.

There is another way that a cheese fondue can kill you. If you are on a particular type of antidepressant drug – a monoamine oxidase inhibitor (MAOI) – then eating cheese is dangerous. A reaction between ingredients in the cheese and the MAOI can push up your blood pressure to dangerous levels, putting you at high risk of a stroke. Drinking alcohol with it increases that risk. So enjoy your cheese fondue, but make sure you don't imbibe unwisely while you do so. And refuse it if you are on an MAOI.

Do our genes determine whether we become alcoholics or not?

Partly, they do. Studies of alcoholics suggest that a substantial proportion of them possess a particular variant of the 'alcohol dehydrogenase' gene that makes them tolerate much more alcohol than other people. That may let them drink more than is healthy without feeling the ill effects that others do. This may be the first step on the rocky road to alcoholism. However, anyone, with any mix of genes, can become alcoholic, suggesting that it is social circumstances rather than basic body biochemistry that matters most of the time.

There is one exception, on the other side of the coin. Some people have a form of another gene, 'aldehyde dehydrogenase' that makes them particularly sensitive to the effects of alcohol. They feel sick and ill after drinking only a small amount. Naturally, they soon learn to avoid more than the minimum of alcohol, and don't become alcoholic. Maybe they are the lucky ones.

Why can't we women drink as much as men before we get liver damage?

Sadly you have a smaller liver than the average man, and

you need much more of yours to deal with your sex hormones. That leaves less capacity to deal with alcohol. It's tough, but proven. Your liver has about two-thirds of the capacity of a man's liver in breaking down alcohol. So your limit is set at about two-thirds of his. There are individual women who can drink more, but that depends on their alcohol dehydrogenase levels. This is the enzyme that breaks down alcohol in the body. Some people make a lot of it, others very little. The more you can produce, the more alcohol you can swallow before you become drunk. Most women use their dehydrogenase to break down their sex hormones – oestrogen and progesterone – which leaves less for the alcohol. So their blood alcohol level builds up faster and stays higher for longer than men's do. Women are something like Japanese men, in that at least half of all Japanese men, and other men in the Far East, make very little alcohol dehydrogenase. As a result they get drunk very quickly on minimal amounts of alcohol. You can tell when they are on the sauce because they turn bright red. And, boy, do they have hangovers the next day.

Why do some people get cancer and others don't, despite smoking just as much or living in the same environment?

Crucial to whether or not you will get cancer of a particular organ is whether or not you have inherited the right or wrong set of genes. Some genes, when 'switched on' by outside influences, can start the process leading to cancer. They are called oncogenes. Other genes protect against cancer. Probably the best known of these is called P53. P53's job is to detect any abnormal change in a cell that might be the start of the cancer process. Once it does so, P53 instructs the cell to 'commit suicide', so that it disappears, and its chemistry is broken down to the basic elements to be circulated away and reused in different ways. The medical name for this process is apoptosis.

Every cell in our bodies contains our version of the P53 gene. If it is damaged in some way, then apoptosis doesn't happen, any cancerous change can continue, and the process towards full-blown cancer can't be stopped. We know that in lung cancer, one of the actions of the chemicals in cigarettes is to damage the P53 gene. We know, too, that in families in which there have been several cases of bowel cancer, many of the sufferers have inherited either a faulty P53 gene or a change in a gene labelled 18qLOH.

So the answer to the question is that it depends on your genetic make-up. Some people are protected against cancer because they don't possess oncogenes. Others are protected because they have a robust P53 system. Yet others are at high risk because they possess oncogenes (they have been detected in people with breast, lung, ovarian and uterine cancers) or because their habits (such as smoking) have destroyed their main anti-cancer defences.

How about the Queen Mum? She smoked like a chimney and lived until she was 101. How do you explain that?

I'm glad you asked that. In the 1980s she allowed her royal warrant to be put on packs of Rothmans cigarettes. At that time I wrote a column for a Scottish Sunday newspaper, and I was furious that the royals should endorse the habit that was killing so many of my patients. So I listed the deaths of the last few Kings of the United Kingdom. Edward VII died of chronic lung failure in 1910, having had a terrible last two years of his life. George V went the same way in 1935, gasping his last breaths, and helped on his way, apparently, by a compassionate royal doctor. Edward VIII died of throat cancer. George VI died of lung cancer and heart disease.

All of their deaths were directly due to their dependence on tobacco. They all put their royal approval on to their favourite brands. Then, of course, there was Princess Margaret...

So I couldn't believe that the Queen Mum approved of

the very material that had killed her husband and was eventually to kill her daughter. My article was waved on the floor of the House of Commons by an anti-smoking MP, and I had my 15 minutes of fame. I don't think I'll be on the Honours List.

So how did the Queen Mum last so long? She was lucky enough to inherit the right genes – and most of the rest of the House of Windsor clearly didn't. You win some, you lose some.

The Amateur Anthropologist

The AA is a perpetual student of life. Interested in the 'bigger picture', Amateur Anthropologists want to know about the fundamentals, not fiddly unimportant things like their own particular health make-up. So they are the opposite of the Neurotic Mother and the Paranoid Party Animal. They want to know about the larger questions in the great scheme of things, and think, quite erroneously, that a GP is likely to have something to offer in the way of answers. They wish to add to the great store of knowledge in their already encyclopaedic brains, and how better to do it than to glean whatever knowledge they can from whichever 'expert' they meet on life's complex way? From the answers I give below, you will quickly realise that the Amateur Anthropologist is chasing moonbeams when he approaches me. That doesn't seem to matter, though, because once he has you in his clutches, he never lets go.

Why are some nations taller than others – for example, Dutch, Zulus, and so on?

This is one of the many questions whose answers are found in the fact that we used to be hunter-gatherers. Go back a few hundred thousand years – up to four million, in fact. Humans lived either on the plains of Africa or in the forests. It was an advantage to be tall if you lived on the grasslands, because you could look over the five-foot-tall grasses and see the sabre-tooth cats coming after you. It was also an advantage to be a speedy runner on two legs. So long legs and upright posture and hands that could throw spears were a bonus. Hence the Zulus and the Ethiopians, Kenyans and so on, all of whom lost the genes for shortness.

On the other hand, if you lived in the jungles, height was a disadvantage in getting through the mess of undergrowth – it was better to be smaller. Hence the pygmies and the Hottentots, who lost the genes for tallness. Tallness may have been an advantage in northern countries, in that the slim tall body structure gives more surface area for body weight, and that allows the skin to take advantage of as much sunlight as it can get. Being fair-skinned helped, too, in allowing the skin to make as much vitamin D as possible throughout the summertime.

As for the Dutch, their being big has a more modern background. They have been big on dairy foods for many centuries, and that has allowed them to grow to their maximum potential. The Finns were similar. Since we Brits began eating more healthily (yes, we have) in the latter half of the 20th century, the average height for adults has grown by more than two inches, in both sexes. We are getting closer to the Dutch and Scandinavians.

How long can we live? Is that ordained from birth, or are we all going to live longer than ever before?

If you want to live for 150 years I have bad news for you. It seems that our lifespan is predictable from birth and there is nothing we can do about it – except change our genetic make-up, and that is a long time in the future, if it is ever possible.

The crucial point is how often our cells can renew themselves. That's the cells of all our organs, from our skin to our gut, our brain, liver and heart, and all the rest. In each organ our cells are constantly renewing themselves – some faster than others. Our gut lining cells and our bone marrow cells (which make our blood cells) 'turn over' faster than our bone cells and nerve cells. But they are all programmed to multiply just so many times, and no more.

Critical to this programme is the telomere. That's a structure at the end of each chromosome. We have 23 pairs of chromosomes, and each time a cell is renewed, the chromosomes line up and divide, to produce two more cells just like their parent. The problem is that, in order to divide, the chromosomes lose a little piece of the telomere. As we age, our telomeres become shorter and shorter, until there is no telomere left. Without a telomere, the cells can't be renewed, and they die – and we die too.

So we could find out precisely how long we are likely to live by measuring the length of our telomeres at birth. The longer they are, the longer we live. Some people are programmed to die in their seventies, some in their nineties. Do you want to know about yours? No, I guessed you don't. As far as I know, no one is routinely measuring telomere length at the moment – but I would be surprised if it didn't happen in the future.

In any case, there is one small drawback to relying on telomere length as a prediction of longevity. When cells renew themselves they sometimes make mistakes, and the new chromosomes aren't perfect. That's one way cancer starts, so you can have a long telomere, yet die earlier than you should have because of a 'transcription error' (the technical name for such mistakes). It's tough that we are programmed to die either of old age, because we run out of chromosome length, or of cancer, because our chromosome replication is faulty. But that's life – and there is plenty of research going on into both problems. Interestingly, I have the impression that the researchers into these problems are a generation older than the usual. I wonder why.

So does the length of our telomeres run in families? Do we inherit the tendency to live a long time from our parents?

It's all up to your father – not your mum. Telomere length seems to pass from father to child (son or daughter), and mum is largely irrelevant. That's the result of Swedish research, but I suppose the Swedes are no different from the rest of us.

They also found that the chromosomes from 'older' sperm (that is, sperm taken from older men) possessed longer telomeres than those from 'young' sperm. So it seems likely that the older your father was when you were conceived, the longer your telomeres will be, and therefore the longer you are likely to live. It's only theory so far, but the science is good. So if you want to predict how long you've got, look at your father's side of the family tree, and forget mum. But remember that there were many influences on life and death in previous generations (and now) that were nothing to do with inheritance. Your father might well have been programmed for a much longer life than he actually had.

Could a man be given injections to make his breasts give milk?

As a father I'd love to have been able to share the breast-feeding duty, but I see difficulties. Yes, it would be possible to give a man injections to produce female-type working breasts that would produce milk. He would need oestrogens and progestins first to develop the breast, then prolactin to switch on the milk. It would almost certainly work, but so far I don't believe it has been tried in human beings.

That's because there's a tiny drawback. Injections of the hormones would have powerful anti-male hormone effects. The would-be breast-feeder would lose his potency and his interest in, and urge for, sex. It would certainly be very effective contraception – the baby couldn't expect a little brother or sister. And there might be a touch of marital discord. But what does that matter, as long as dad does his fair share of feeding?

Why do women live longer?

What if I said that we men look after your every whim, protect you from stress and worry all your lives, and die early from the extra burden that places on us? Would you believe it? Probably not, but I gave it a try. Sadly, we poor males usually die younger than you robust females because we are born with a big disadvantage. That Y-chromosome that differentiates us from you carries little else but sex chromatin (the protein that determines that we have the dangly bits). It's a tiny apology for a decent chromosome. On the other hand you have two X chromosomes, fully resplendent with a host of goodies other than their sex proteins. That gives females the edge in all sorts of ways – you have extra strands to your immune systems and you are immune from a host of illnesses. And it is that X chromosome advantage which probably explains why in general you live longer than us – if you manage to survive into old age – by about five years. Some of the extra years depend, too, on lifestyle rather than inheritance.

Marriage seems to help both sexes to live longer: married men live on average seven years longer than bachelors, and married women two years longer than spinsters. That tends to suggest that men get a bit more out of married life than women. But if you really want, as a woman, to live longer, join a convent, the earlier in life the better. Particularly in Minnesota. A 2006 study has highlighted Minnesota nuns as the longest-living community. Maybe it's because they laugh a lot. Another aspect of long life, apparently, is a good sense of humour, and a lot of laughing. You think that might be strange for nuns? Not in my experience – I've had the great privilege of looking after two communities of nuns, and they are an absolute hoot.

Why do I keep gathering blue fluff in my navel?

Navels are much-neglected organs. Their only known use ends at birth. So people tend to ignore them, so much so that they gather detritus, often over many years. Of course, people shower and bathe, but when soaping their tummies, they often forget to clean out that particular nook (or is it a cranny?). As the years pass, the hollow fills with the solid remnants of shed skin, sweat, material from underclothing, even bits of soap – and they can set as hard as a stone. A major job of junior surgeons when 'preparing' the skin of the abdomen for surgery is to dig out these bits of stone, to prevent infection spreading from them into the wound during the operation. We even have a name for it – umbilical lithotomy – and it's been known for the bigger ones to be used as a 'catch' question in surgical Finals examinations. Sometimes you can get an infection in the navel with a germ that produces a blue colony. There's one called Pseudomonas pyocyaneus. It's a lovely blue colour, but not a very nice germ. An antiseptic soap should fix it.

Why does asparagus make my pee smell?

It's not just asparagus. Eating quite a few vegetables makes your pee smell. Surely you've noticed, too, that it smells after eating seafoods – like shellfish or oily fish. Beer isn't odourless, either, when you get rid of its chemical remnants. That's what these smells are – chemical remnants of the substances that made your food so tasty in the first place. Their odour isn't necessarily so attractive after your gut, liver and kidneys have had a go at them. It's all about how you process what you eat after you have digested it. Your liver turns it into the substances you need – proteins and fats, and combinations of them, along with glucose – for your continuing healthy existence. Necessarily the process produces some waste products, and the more volatile of them, that are soluble in water, are concentrated, then excreted by your kidneys.

Turn your mind back to your schooldays, and to all those smells, fair and foul, your chemistry teacher used to create in the organic chemistry lab. They came from aldehydes and ketones – chemicals that drifted through the air like perfumes or farts. When our livers have dealt with asparagus, garlic, prawns and the like, aldehydes and ketones are what the kidney has to process into our urine. Dissolved in urine inside the body, they don't reach our nostrils. Once released into the air of your toilet pan, that's a different matter.

It's not a bad thing that the urine smells. Sometimes a different smell in the urine is the initial sign of a disease – which is why doctors in the past made a thing out of smelling pee. The classic is the sweet smell of acetone (like pear drops) that may be the first sign that you have diabetes. So if your urine starts to smell odd, and you haven't eaten anything unusual, it isn't a bad thing to let your doctor have a sample. Luckily we don't have to smell (or taste!) the stuff any more – we have sophisticated biochemical tests that will do the job for us.

Why do some people have a third nipple?

In the first few weeks of our human development after conception, we go through a host of changes. One of them is to develop a 'nipple line' that runs from above to below on each side of the chest and abdomen, roughly from the middle of the collarbone down to the middle of the groin.

Spaced fairly evenly along that line is a series of nipples, perhaps four to six on each side. As we grow further and begin to develop a more human shape, the extra nipple cells obey an inbuilt message to 'commit suicide' in much the same way as the cells in a tadpole's tail do when they develop into a frog (it's the same process, called apoptosis). In most people, only the nipples that are in the position they will be in an adult survive. But nothing in nature is written in stone, so for a small number of us, a few extra nipples remain resistant to apoptosis. Hence the occasional retention of one, two or even more extra nipples. I don't know of anyone, however, whose extra nipples ever produced milk or were associated with a recognizable female breast.

Does your hat size relate to the size of your brain?

No, it doesn't. I can vouch for that personally. I have a relatively big head, with a hat size of $7^3/4$ inches. Being an arrogant male, I obviously thought that this meant I had a large brain. Until I was in a car crash and needed a skull X-ray. It showed that my skull bones were much thicker than usual, the extra bone explaining my larger cranium. My brain size was depressingly average. Then again, brain size isn't important – see the answer to the next question.

Are men's brains bigger than women's?

On average, yes, but that's not the important measurement. There are considerable differences between male and female human brains. You men are not going to like this answer, but here goes.

With apologies to Hercule Poirot, we men must admit that women have more 'little grey cells' in the front of the brain (the 'frontal cortex') and have more complex and more numerous communications between the grey cells than men. Women's brains even have a higher blood flow through the frontal cortex than men's. All these differences favour the fact that, in this part of the brain, women have the advantage. The frontal cortex is the part of the brain you use to form judgments and make decisions. So the female brain is more efficient, and better all round.

Sorry, gentlemen, there's no argument about that.

What is the origin of the old wives' tale that redheads smell different?

The idea that redheads smell different from other women (no one cares about how redheaded men smell) comes from the Frenchman Augustin Galopin, who wrote *Le*

Parfum de la Femme in 1886. He had the weird theory that redheaded women had the strongest scent of all women, and that they smelled of amber. (Brunettes, he claimed, smelled of ebony, and blondes had a much fainter smell of amber or violets.)

Now that puzzles me. Amber is a fossil, for goodness sake! How can it have a smell, and how can redheads smell like it? Yet here we are, 120 years later, still discussing the subject.

To put the record straight, redheads differ biochemically from the rest of us in only one way: they can't make melanin in their skins. They have a variation in the gene that makes melanin, so that they make a red pigment instead, called pheomelanin. It makes them more than normally susceptible to skin cancer, but it has nothing to do with their body odour. The composition of their sweat – from the armpits, groins or the rest of the body – is no different from that of non-redheads. Maybe the redheads you know buy a different range of perfumes and body lotions?

On the subject of BO, why do I sometimes smell awful and other times smell fine?

Body odour is made up of a mixture of things. What you

ate last night matters – volatile substances in garlic and onions pass into your sweat. Have you been emotionally (sexually excited? angry? anxious?) involved recently? If so, then the glands in the armpits, groins and the small of your back may have been overactive, and they produce more pungent aromas than normal skin sweat. Have you washed regularly? If you haven't, then bacteria and fungi can produce pongs after a while. In an ordinary day, with a non-Mediterranean meal the previous evening, no obvious excitement and a shower before going out, sweat doesn't smell at all. It is only a salt and water solution, after all.

Is there such a state as suspended animation? Could people be kept alive indefinitely with no heartbeat and no breathing, then brought back to life, undamaged?

The immediate, unthinking response to this question is, of course, 'no'. But hang on a minute. In January 2000, the *Lancet* reported the case of Anna Bagenholm. She had fallen head first through a crack in river ice when cross-country skiing, and was not found and brought out of the water until 80 minutes later. Her body temperature was more than 20 degrees below normal. There was no audible heartbeat and no perceptible breathing movement. She was taken by helicopter to hospital, where her blood was removed, warmed up and fed back into her veins. After 60 days in intensive care she made a full recovery with no long-term ill effects.

Was this a one-off, a freak survival? Or is it a mechanism that exists in all of us? Hasan Alam, a trauma surgeon at Massachusetts General Hospital, thinks it could be used to save many lives. He has taken the body temperature of anaesthetised pigs down to 10 degrees Celsius (the normal is 37) removed all their blood, operated on multiple serious injuries while they were in this apparently dead state, then transfused back the animals' own warmed blood. When their body temperatures reached 25 degrees, their hearts started again, and a seemingly dead animal came back to normal life.

Dr Alam sees this as a step to helping very badly injured trauma patients through their first few hours. Much more intricate and longer repairs are possible if the surgeon is not pressurised by the need to keep the patient well oxygenated and supplied with blood – in an average severe trauma case it is common for the patient to need transfusion with more than three times their whole body's blood volume. He reckons the best temperature to maintain full suspended animation is around 10 degrees. Below five degrees the body's cells start to die off. He hopes to do human trials of his pig technique soon, but he has an unusual difficulty. The best patients for the trials would be people who have lost a lot of blood, are badly injured, and who will die very quickly under normal circumstances. By definition they will not be able to give their full consent to be trial subjects. Yet such consent is essential for all new surgical research. For Dr Alam's research team it is a catch-22, unless the whole community agrees in advance to take part, much like organ donors do today.

Can using your brain really make you more intelligent?

Why do you think London taxi drivers are so smart? They are never at a loss for intelligent conversation, and one of them was the UK's *Mastermind* champion. It's probably due to having to acquire 'The Knowledge'. It takes several years and a lot of memory training to pass this test before they can become a professional driver in London.

Dr Eleanor Maguire and her team at University College, who have made a special study of London cabbies, showed that the average cabby's brain has a larger hippocampus than normal. Even more convincing, the longer they had been driving, the bigger their hippocampuses (or should that be hippocampi? – I don't know). As the hippocampus is heavily involved in memory and reasoning, this is a good pointer that training the brain in difficult memory tasks does make you brighter. I must admit that on my visits to London I have always enjoyed the banter in the taxi. Compare it with, say, drivers in other capital cities, who don't have to go through the same rigorous training. Dare I mention New York?

Is being left-handed an advantage or a disadvantage over being right-handed?

Two generations ago, it was a distinct disadvantage. Teachers forced left-handed children to use their right hands, to the point of being cruel to them – although there were obvious practical disadvantages: writing with a left hand in ink usually meant you smudged the page as your hand followed the ink across the page instead of leading it. Thankfully that prejudice has gone and left-handers are allowed to develop naturally in all the manual skills they need.

If the question means do left-handed people have a different type of brain from right-handed ones, then the answer is probably 'no'. The latest research divides people not into left- or right-handed, but into 'strong-handers' or 'weak-handers'. You can tell which you are by noting which hand you use for everyday tasks such as writing, drawing, throwing, using scissors, a toothbrush, a knife without a fork, and a spoon. Do you use the same hand as the upper one on a yard brush or spade, as the one you use to hold a match when you strike it or the lid of a box when opening it? Mark down for each of these activities which hand you 'always' or 'usually' use. Strong-handed people will mark the same one (whether right or left) for them all, and mostly as 'always'. Mixed-handed people will switch hands around for different tasks. Interestingly, on this scoring system, only around 2 per cent of the population are strong left-handers.

Studies of handedness have dispelled the myth, for example, that left-handed people are more creative and right-handers are more logical: they apparently don't differ very much. However, there are differences between the strong-handers on both sides and the mixed-handers. Mixed-handers appear to have longer and more accurate memories than strong-handers. If they are musical, then mixed-handers gravitate more to stringed instruments and strong-handers to drums and keyboards. Some brain researchers tentatively suggest that this is because mixed-handers have a stronger connection (it is a structure called the corpus callosum) between the two halves of the brain. They can therefore deal better with tasks that need the co-ordination of the whole brain. Other researchers are less convinced: they say that social and cultural influences on people are far greater than the mere size of the connections between the two halves of the brain in determining their character and their skills.

I wonder if anyone has compared, say, violinists and percussionists, for memory loss in their old age? It might settle the argument. I've not heard of anyone actually doing such a study, but it would make a good PhD thesis.

Does 'SAD' (Seasonal Affective Disorder) really exist, and does sunshine cure it?

Every GP will tell you that the depression workload rises in January (after the Christmas and New Year holiday) and goes on until the spring. If the weather in spring and early summer stays rotten, with a lot of cloud and rain, then SAD will worsen.

I remember one May in which it rained every day. In all my years in practice I had the highest consultation rate for depression in that month – beating every January and February by a country mile. But don't ask me about the lack of sun and depression. Ask the good people of Rattenberg in the Tyrol. This village is situated deep in a valley, with little sun penetrating all year round. Currently, in an attempt to lift their collective spirits, they are placing giant mirrors on the hills on the opposite side of the valley to reflect the sun down towards them. The mirrors will follow the sun, so that the villagers (who are presumably miserable at the moment) will bask in it from dawn to dusk. Will they suddenly become joyous Austrians? Will their doctors have a happier time, too? As a colleague I hope so.

How did patients survive operations in the days before anaesthetic was invented?

The secret was in the surgeons being so fast that the operation was finished almost before the patient had time to react to it. It is said that during an operation performed by one Professor Langenbeck, a German surgeon in the early 19th century, one of his colleagues turned away from the operating table for a moment to take a pinch of snuff (imagine that in today's theatres) and completely missed a shoulder amputation. There's the apocryphal story, too, of Professor Ashley Cooper, operating in England at about the same time as Professor Langenbeck in Germany. In amputating one man's leg through the mid-thigh, with one circular sweep of his curved amputating knife, he 'cut off the tail of the coat of one assistant and two fingers of another'.

Curious George

Happily, the relationship between doctors and other people's children is a fairly formal one. In the surgery, most children who are there to be seen are quiet, a little frightened, and shy. They are no bother, and by the end of the meeting doctor and child are usually good friends. It's their siblings – little brother or sister – who know they aren't in for questions, examinations or, worse, tests, who are the menace. They have to be present because mum can't pass them off to someone else (it's often unsurprising that they can't) and they can run riot in the room.

'What's this for?' they ask, having got hold of (you don't know how, as you have been examining their sibling's sore ear) a vaginal speculum. After blood pressure machines, stethoscopes, patella hammers and piles of notes have gone crashing to the floor, the little angel turns to you and asks: 'How did my little brother get into mummy's tummy?' And follows it up with: 'And how is he going to get out?' You know that he knows perfectly well the answers to both questions, and that he is only asking in order to watch you squirm. But you smile sweetly, don't answer, and make the rest of the consultation as short as possible. It's then that you want to demonstrate exactly what you could do with that speculum. But you forbear because you quite like being a doctor, really. The plus side to Curious George is that sometimes he does actually ask questions that make you think.

What are bogies made of?

I suppose I must answer this question, though it offends my literary sensibilities. Nasal mucus, to give bogies their correct title, is the result of a titanic battle between the bad guys (bacteria and viruses) and the good guys (our wonderful immune system) that goes on almost every day of our lives. We breathe in droplets from other people's coughs and sneezes, upon which the bad guys are hitching rides, and they settle on the surfaces inside our nose. The nose is amazingly efficient in 'sweeping' the air inside it on to the 'brushes' that protrude into its passages – so much so that very few droplets and dust particles can pass through it directly into the lungs. When they land on nasal surfaces, our first-line defensive cells produce mucus – a sort of goo – within which there are chemicals that recognise and coat the germs. They also send a chemical message to marshal second-line defensive cells to come to the spot and deal with the invaders. The cells recognise the enemy from their coating of chemicals, and start to engulf them. In the fight, there are casualties on both sides, leaving the mess of dead cells and germs to be mopped up by the mucus.

Bogies are this detritus of a battle you probably didn't know was going on daily inside your nose. Only when it becomes a terrifying war zone – as in a cold – do you feel the consequences in a sore and itchy nose.

What is it that makes us suddenly have a shiver, like when 'someone walks over our grave'?

Have you seen a cat's hair bristle – say, when it sees a dog nearby? All the fur stands on end, at an exact right angle to the skin surface. Or noticed how fat a bird's body looks in the coldest days of winter, because the feathers are all fluffed out? Our sudden 'shiver' is a remnant of those responses: they go back in our ancestry to the times when we were struggling small rat-like furry mammals trying to keep out of the way of the dinosaurs. And maybe even before that.

Of course, we don't have fur, but we do have very fine hair all over the body that you can hardly see. When we are relaxed, the hairs lie flat against our skin. At the base of each hair is a muscle whose job is to pull its hair upright, so that it stands up, like the cat's fur and the bird's feathers. In the distant past, when we were covered in thick hair, this was a great defence mechanism. The erect fur made us look bigger than we were to deceive enemies. Probably more important, the thicker covering trapped warm air against the skin, protecting us from the cold. When we are cold today, we still get goose pimples – each goose pimple is one of the muscles raising its remnant of hair.

So why do we still have these spine-chilling shivering fits, now that the hairs are too small to serve a purpose? We still have the nerve system that goes into action when the body perceives a threat – the sympathetic nervous system. And branches of the sympathetic nerves serve each one of the goose-pimple muscles. So when we have had a slight surprise, or are hit suddenly by a cold draught, or we perceive consciously or unconsciously that we are facing some sort of primeval threat, our sympathetic system still goes into action. One of these actions is to raise our goose pimples, all of them, almost in one action, so that we feel a flood of hairs rising down our backs. We are just like the cat seeing the dog. It takes only seconds, and when the stimulus is over, the nerves return to their baseline activity.

Why do our teeth chatter when we are cold?

That's different from the 'someone is walking over my grave' scenario. When our body temperature drops, we need to generate heat to keep it at the very narrow range of one degree around 37 degrees. Making the muscles contract and relax quickly does that very efficiently – hence the shivering – and the big jaw muscles that cause teeth to chatter are perfect for the job.

Why do we cry?

You have obviously never had the discomfort of a dry eye, or you wouldn't ask this question. For your eye to function, its surface must be moist all the time. So our tear glands above and behind the outside angle of the upper eyelids must constantly produce tears to keep the surface covered in watery fluid. The eyelids blink to make sure that the tears are distributed over the whole eye. Then the tears are drained away into the nose by another duct, the entrance to which is on the inner edge of the lower eyelid, next to the nose. If your tears dry up, the eye becomes red and very sore, and prone to infection. In fact, Sir Alexander Fleming was researching the antibiotic properties of tears (a substance called lysozyme) before he came across penicillin.

We all know what makes us cry – pain, grief, sadness, anxiety, all the unpleasant emotions. That's the easy part of the question answered. But what the purpose or benefit of crying is in such circumstances is more difficult to understand. The physiological answer might include that the production of tears is the result of stimulation of the sympathetic nervous system, which is on duty at full pelt in such circumstances, so that tears are just an accidental accompaniment to the rest of the reactions going on elsewhere in the body. The psychologist would go further and suggest that crying is a very personal outward show of the emotion that you feel in the circumstances in which you find yourself. If that is seen by your friends and family it is understood to be something that needs pity, sympathy, and attention. It is the perfect physiological reaction to elicit comfort at a time when it is most needed. How this started must have happened thousands of years ago, when the human face began to be able to show emotion.

If I have big ears, will I hear better?

What's the point of ears fixed to the sides of our heads? They're not like the ears of some animals, such as bats, which use them for direction-finding. A few people can wiggle their ears, but not to any useful purpose. And they play only a very minor part in collecting sound waves – people born with very small ears or with almost no external ear at all can usually still hear well. Once the sound has reached the earhole it is then channelled along a tube towards the outer eardrum, where the process of hearing really begins. The outside shape of the ears makes no difference to that process.

A good example of why it doesn't is found in marine animals. Seals have no external ears – sea lions have quite prominent ones. There's no evidence that lack of ears makes seals less able to hear than sea lions. We understand very well what happens once the sound reaches the eardrum – it is magnified by the three bones inside the middle ear, then collected and sorted in the inner ear, which turns the sound into electrical activity along the auditory nerve to the brain, which then interprets the sound accordingly. The external ear plays very little part in that process. So I must conclude that the most important function of my external ears is merely to hold my glasses in place.

Why do I feel a bit sick if I put my finger in my belly button?

This is a new one on me, but there are possible reasons. John L Sullivan and Harry Houdini, if they were here, might be able to throw light on the answer. But they're well past their sell-by dates now.

My own feeling about this relationship between navel manipulation (for want of a better word) and feeling sick is that you must be stimulating your solar plexus. This is a bunch of nerves lying in the back of the abdomen just behind your navel. It controls the main movements of your gut and the process of digestion. Stimulate it in the wrong way and the gut muscles shut down. That can certainly make you feel nauseous.

What was that about Sullivan and Houdini?

John L Sullivan was a world boxing champion in the late 19th century. Until he came on the scene, boxers concentrated on hitting the chest and the chin. He developed the solar plexus punch. A sharp punch to the navel caused the gut to become paralysed and the blood vessels inside the whole abdomen dilated suddenly – so that Sullivan's unfortunate opponent no longer had any blood flow back from the abdomen to the heart. The result was a total inability to fight on, and a win for the champion by a knockout.

Since John L's time, all boxers are trained to defend themselves against a solar plexus punch, by keeping their abdominal muscles tense throughout their fights.

And Houdini?

Houdini knew all about the solar plexus and how to defend himself against a punch in the abdomen – so much so that he threw a challenge to anyone to try to knock him out, or even hurt him, using a punch to the belly. He put up a big prize to the person who could do it. Many people tried, even using hammers and mallets, but he was always ready for them, and shrugged off the blow.

Until one day, when he had just eaten in a restaurant and was preparing to leave the table. Catching him unawares, a young man punched him in the navel while his muscles were relaxed and his stomach was full of food. The punch pole-axed him and ruptured his gut. He died three days later of peritonitis.

The Alternative Medicine Addict

This party pest is, I'm afraid, almost always female. She isn't badgering you to get advice from you – not at all. She is there to give you a piece of advice, and of her mind, too. To her, doctors have been seduced away from the true path by the pharmaceutical industry and the orthodoxy of the medical establishment, and have forgotten the healing ways of mother nature. Anything 'natural' must be better, by definition, than anything 'chemical'. So she sticks to herbs, a vegan diet, and all the current alternative fashions. We get a diatribe on homeopathy, acupuncture, iridology, reflexology, Reiki, Taoism, colonic irrigation, the wholeness of things, and the benefit of prayer to mother earth, the sun or any mystic (preferably eastern) deity. She talks at length about the benefits of echinacea, St John's wort, gingko biloba, feverfew, evening primrose oil, green-lipped mussel, and vitamins A, B, C, D, E and K. If there were others she would talk about them, too. She knows as much about their function in the body as she does about the engineering of a jumbo jet and how to fly it, but that doesn't stop her pontificating about them.

She talks of 'energy fields', 'vibrations' and 'auras', and uses crystals, magnets and pendula to divine and even cure illnesses. Never mind that everything she claims blatantly contradicts the laws of physics – she can cure any ailment provided you think the right way. And, crucially, if her methods don't work, it's your fault for not believing in them, never hers.

It's no use explaining to her that the developments in modern medicine over the past 30 years have saved many millions of people from dying early of high blood pressure, heart attacks and strokes, stomach ulcers, infections, cancers, leukaemias, lymphomas, diabetes, forms of arthritis, and have helped people tolerate and survive many inherited and other diseases. And that we had her alternative ways of treating people for thousands of years without them making a scrap of difference to life expectancy and quality.

She won't listen. So I suggest that the next time she goes on holiday she should try an alternative airline that builds planes and trains on the same lines as the alternative medicine promoters produce their cure-alls. She doesn't think it funny, and walks away, with a sharp remark that I'm not taking her seriously. Actually I do take people like her very seriously. From time to time over the years I have found them dangerous and interfering in the progress of very sick people, sometimes to their great detriment. So I'm not upset that she has stormed off in a huff.

Is organic food always better for you than non-organic?

No. Not in my opinion – let me explain. First, plants are not entirely 'organic'. They actually feed on inorganic materials. That is, their roots pick up inorganic – not organic – minerals from the soil around them. They absorb potassium, sodium, magnesium, selenium, nitrate, sodium, ammonium, phosphate, carbonate, silicate and a host of other minerals direct from their surroundings. They don't care if these goodies have been delivered to them in manure or in bags of fertiliser: in fact, they don't have a mechanism whereby they can choose to differentiate between them. If magnesium is in the soil around the roots, then they will pick it up regardless, whether or not it has got there through a so-called 'organic' system. The end result is the same. The carrot will still be a carrot with the same chemical structure and offer the same nutritional value whether it has been grown organically or not.

I can understand that people are frightened that non-organically grown vegetables and fruits may have residues of pesticides and weedkillers in them and that they might harm their health. On the other hand, organic vegetables and fruit may have more parasites in them. No one has yet worked out the benefits against the drawbacks in any long-term study – which should involve analysing samples of tissues from people who have lived entirely organically for years and comparing them with the same from people who have lived off normal supermarket produce. I would bet that the organic industry won't take the risk of doing so – in case the results are on the wrong side for them.

In the meantime, since we as a population took to eating foods prepared with modern methods there has been no rise in ill health due directly to choosing them instead of organic foods. The exception is that we eat too much, and become obese, but that's separate from the organic-versus-non-organic argument.

As far as I understand the economics of farming and eating, I believe that we need to feed the world, and we need to grow enough crops to do so. Could we do that entirely with organic farming methods?

Are coffee enemas worthwhile?

Why on earth would anyone want to put coffee into his or her bowel? The end of the large bowel isn't designed for digesting things. It's an organ of excretion, and a pretty efficient one, too, if you leave it in peace to do its job. Its lining wasn't meant to come into contact with coffee. Things come out of it – it's not made for things going into it. Just the thought of putting coffee into the rectum, then cleaning up and washing the tubing afterwards should put anyone off doing it or receiving it. Were you thinking of administering it yourself? Do you add milk and sugar? We don't have taste buds in our bottoms, and for a very good reason, considering the material inside them. At what temperature is the coffee on insertion? It's nonsense. If you want the benefit of coffee, why not just drink it?

Can drinking soya milk be bad for you?

Soya isn't any different from other manufactured foods, in that most people can eat it and it will provide the standard nutrients (proteins, fats and carbohydrates) that we get from a host of others, such as dairy products. It's just that the detailed structures of these foodstuffs differ from those of other vegetables. Most of the time that doesn't matter, because our digestive system breaks them down and transfers their basic 'building blocks' on to our livers, which then build them up into our own types of proteins, fats and carbohydrates. Problems arise only when the immune system in some people (fairly few, luckily) sees the soya material as 'foreign' enough to need special treatment, and reacts fairly violently against it. This can cause digestive upsets and other vague illness. So for some people soya is a nuisance, much in the same way as milk is for others.

People who react badly to milk have gut pains and bloating because they don't possess the enzymes in the gut to break down the milk sugar lactose. So they turn to soya, which has no lactose. That's a reasonable step to take. However, I can't really reconcile that with what happens around the Mediterranean. A much higher proportion of people living around the Med are lactose intolerant than we in northern Europe are. Yet I haven't heard of many Italians, Greeks and Spaniards turning to soya instead. They enjoy delicious food, with very little milk. Could it be that Mediterranean cooking is perfectly suited to us, without the need to turn to soya?

Why do people in health shops always look so unhealthy?

Why do you think they went there in the first place? Healthy people don't need to go into health shops. If you are already healthy, there's nothing you can take to make you more healthy.

Does milk really give you cancer?

Who would have thought that anyone would even think up this question – until 2006? This is the scare put forward by Heather Mills McCartney and her friends at the Vegetarian and Vegan Society. They claimed in May 2006 that dairy products are responsible for almost all the ills that beset modern human beings, among them (I quote from their press release) 'certain cancers, heart disease, diabetes, osteoporosis and obesity'. I'll name her supporters, so that you can make your own judgment: they are Professor T Colin Campbell of Cornell University; Professor Jane Plant, described as 'top scientist'; and Juliet Gellatley, founder of Viva, the largest vegetarian and vegan organisation in Europe. Look up their work on the internet if you wish, but understand that they have one desire in common – to get rid of all farm animals, and to persuade everyone to become at least vegetarian, and preferably vegan. I prefer to base my judgments on the safety and benefits of milk on the work of people who are less motivated by such personal beliefs. At the moment I can see absolutely no reason to abandon milk as a nutritious food.

Can the oestrogen in modern water supplies make us impotent?

As far as I understand it, the problem with oestrogens is not that they are in our drinking water, but that they are in our sewage effluent. (They are the consequence of women excreting the hormones ingested in their contraceptive tablets.) The sewage works do not filter them out of the final water effluent, so they reach our rivers, where fish and other water creatures absorb them. That's bad for the male fish, because they turn into hapless semi-females and can no longer father little fishes.

However, oestrogens in drinking water are another matter. They shouldn't be there, as waterworks must ensure that the drinking water is free from such contaminants. I've asked our local watermen, and they are unaware of any problem with our water. And I haven't noticed any lack of interest in sex among our young male population – rather the reverse.

However, there's no doubt that if even tiny amounts of oestrogens get into a water supply, sex problems will follow: young men will grow breasts and find their accoutrements shrinking and flopping. Neither they nor their partners will find this satisfactory. How do I know this? Back in the 1960s when men first worked on the production lines for the contraceptive pill, they inhaled tiny amounts of the pill powder. They changed in just the way I described above. The women production line workers were also badly affected. Many of them became infertile – they were inhaling enough of the dust each month for it to act as a contraceptive.

The pharmaceutical firms had to develop vacuum systems on the production lines and protective clothing for the operatives to shield them from even the smallest bit of contamination – and things went back to normal for the men and women. So the tiniest amount of oestrogen in drinking water might have serious consequences for the general population.

Does taking probiotic yogurt drinks every day improve your health?

Amazingly, it might! The idea of probiotic yogurts is that

the bacteria in them are similar to those that first exist in a breast-feeding baby's gut, and that are linked with protection against inflammatory bowel disease. They are also responsible for the loose motions that every parent who has ever changed a nappy knows. One doubt raised by the experts is how the 'good bacteria' in the yogurts get past the acid in the stomach without being destroyed. As proteins, they should in theory be digested before they reach the large bowel, which is where they 'do their work'. However, enough of them do seem to survive to change the bowel movements in the right direction, according to their users. But after that it is difficult to judge what difference they make to a person's general health.

Swedish researchers say they have the answer. They showed that people who take probiotics have fewer days off work than those who don't, mainly because they have fewer stomach and digestive complaints. They say that this is not because people who take them are less likely to take time off in any case, but it is difficult to prove this. The jury is still out on their conclusions.

The French pride themselves on their 'natural' health service – but when I go to France and get ill, I seem to be prescribed more pills and potions than I'd ever get in England.

The French have always had a love for medicines that far exceeds our own. The French equivalent of our National Health Service consistently recorded that French doctors prescribe between two and three times as many medicines as we do. The French national bill for pharmaceuticals is at least twice as high as ours, per head. They don't see a contradiction between 'prescription' medicine and 'natural' treatments, feeling that they complement each other. We have been traditionally more wary of what we call 'polypharmacy' (prescribing several different medicines together), but we appear to be catching up with our closest neighbours. It's not just the French who spend a fortune on medicines; look at the costs in Germany (higher still) and in the United States (astronomical). The Americans are trying to change this, with each state establishing 'Managed Care Medicine' in which doctors are being restricted to prescribing from a rigid list of drugs drawn up by 'experts'. It is causing a lot of argument, but rising costs are bound to make this common everywhere in the near future – even in France.

Why can't you take St John's wort when you are on the pill?

People tend to think that if a medicine is just a herb, it's safer and has fewer serious side effects than a prescription drug. That's just pure wrong. If a medicine is effective, say, against depression, as is claimed for St John's wort, then it must be causing a chemical change in the body (in fact, the brain) in the same way as do standard prescription antidepressants. However, St John's wort doesn't just act on the brain. In the liver it 'switches on' the enzymes that the liver produces to break down the hormones in the contraceptive pill. That means the sex hormones in the pill are destroyed faster than usual, probably well before the day is out, leaving you unprotected against ovulation, and therefore conception. So if you combine St John's wort with the pill, you risk becoming pregnant.

But this 'interaction' with the contraceptive pill is only the tip of the St John's wort iceberg. Here's the list in the *British National Formulary* (our 'bible' for prescribing) of the drugs whose actions are altered, blocked or heightened by St John's wort – it's an impressive list for a 'herb':

- Antibacterials – erythromycin (not during and for two weeks after St John's wort)
- Anticoagulants – reduces the effects of warfarin
- Antidepressants – greatly increased effects and side effects
- Anti-epileptics – reduces their effects
- Antimalarials – reduces their protection against malaria

- Anti-psychotic drugs (given for schizophrenia and mania) – reduces the effect
- Antivirals – The *BNF* lists 10 antivirals (used mainly for HIV and herpes) whose blood levels are reduced by St John's wort
- Barbiturates – reduces their effects
- Heart drugs – reduces the effects of digoxin, important in controlling a heart rhythm
- Anti-cancer and post-transplant anti-rejection drugs – reduces their efficiency
- Anti-asthma drugs – reduces their effects.

There are even others with complex purposes for particular illnesses that I've left out.

If there's one preparation that shows how important it is to know all about herbal medicines, and to treat them just like prescription drugs, it is St John's wort.

What was that thing that Gwyneth Paltrow had done with the cups on her back after the birth of Apple. I am eight months pregnant; do I need it?

No, unless you fancy going into labour with a series of hot, red lumps and even blisters all over your back. You are describing 'cupping', a medieval practice involving putting a heated cup or glass rim down on your skin. It has to be hot enough to hurt you.

The principle is as wacky as the result. A thousand years or so ago, when doctors knew nothing about the circulation or even the basic principles of health or disease, they dreamed up dozens of daft ways of treating (duping?) their patients. They bled them, they poulticed them, they 'scoured' them (causing terrible diarrhoea) and generally gave them a terrible time. Read the accounts of the death of Charles II if you want to know how awful the doctors of the time were, and of the many terrible treatments he had to endure before they finally managed to finish him off. He must have envied his father's quick clean death on the block.

One of these treatments was cupping. Doctors thought that by raising the skin up in a lump they were somehow improving their patients' circulation and making them better. The patients felt better when the cupping was stopped, for sure, because it was painful during the treatment and uncomfortable for several hours afterwards. They had to believe 'there's no gain without pain' to endure it. Not many came back for seconds. So, no, you don't need to follow Miss Paltrow's example. The great and the good don't always get the best.

What astounds me is that, in the 21st century, people are still willing to undergo such treatments when there is absolutely no scientific, medical, logical or any other reason for them. Does each new generation never learn from the mistakes of the past?

Quiz

Have you ever considered what your doctor might think of you as a patient? Do you make his/her heart sink or face light up when you enter the surgery? Here's a quiz that should give you pause for thought. It separates the dream patient from the doctor's worst nightmare. Add up your score as you answer the questions – and then see yourself as your doctor sees you.

1. Have you ever put on a ra-ra skirt, fishnets and high heels to visit your doctor?

Count 0 for no, 3 points for yes. If yes and you are over 60, count double. If you are male of any age, multiply by 10.

2. How many of the following do you take every day? Evening primrose oil, betacarotene, vitamins A, B, C, D, E or K, fish oil capsules, zinc, gingko biloba, green-lipped mussel, St John's wort.

Count 1 point for each (including 1 for each vitamin). If more than three multiply by three, if more than five, multiply by 10.

3. How thick are your medical notes?

Count 0 for less than half an inch, 1 for half an inch to two inches, 4 for over two inches, and 10 if they cover half a shelf.

4. How many times have you brought a magazine article or internet download about your illnesses to your doctor?

Count 0 for never, then 1 for each time. Multiply by 10 if over three times.

5. How many different out-of-date (never taken) prescribed medicines do you still have in your bathroom cabinet?

Count 1 for each, and multiply by 10 if over five.

6. How often have you reported that a prescribed medicine has made you sick, given you side effects

or given you an allergy?
Count 0 for never or only once. Count 2 points for each occasion after that. Multiply by 20 if over five times.

7. How often have you come for a normal-length appointment with your doctor and asked about more than two health problems?
Count 1 point for each time and 10 for more than three times.

8. Have you ever written out a list of complaints you want to talk about in your consultation?
If never, or if you asked for a longer appointment, count 0. If you didn't ask for a longer appointment, count 1. If more than once, count 1 point for each time, and then add 2 points for each item on the list. If you score 10 or more on this initial count, multiply by five.

9. When your consultation seems to be over, and you have got as far as the door, have you ever turned and said (like Lieutenant Columbo) 'Oh, and another thing, doctor...'?
Count 10 points for doing this once, and 20 points for each subsequent time you have done it.

10. Do you possess your own set of medical notes

and X-rays at home, and insist on discussing them with your doctor whenever you see him/her?

0 points if you don't, 10 points if you do.

11. Your doctor has prescribed a medicine for you, but your sister/cousin/sibling/spouse says that it isn't the right medicine/is the wrong dose/gave them an allergy or severe side effect/won't do any good. What do you do?

You take no heed of them – 0 points. You return to the doctor with their fears – 1 point. You stop taking them immediately because you have more trust in these non-medical people than your doctor – 10 points.

12. Has your doctor ever asked you to stop smoking, and you haven't?

Count 2 points for the first time, 5 for the second time and 50 points for the third or more. Count minus 10 points if you have never smoked, and minus 5 points if you DID stop the first time you were asked.

13. When the bird flu scare started, did you insist on you and your family being given a prescription for Tamiflu?

0 points if no, 5 points if you did.

14. How many times have you asked for a second

opinion from a doctor other than your GP/ consultant?

If never or once, count 0 points. If twice or more, count 3 points for each time. Multiply by 20 if five times or more.

15. Do you think 'natural medicines' are safer and more effective than modern prescription medicines?

0 points if you think they are not, 2 points if you are doubtful, 10 points if you think they are.

16. As well as visiting your doctor, how many of the following do you also see regularly (without telling him/her)? Your homeopath, osteopath, chiropractor, acupuncturist, reflexologist, iridologist, astrologer, colonic irrigationist, Reiki practitioner, herbalist, crystal therapist, faith healer, hot stone practitioner?

Count 0 points if none, and 2 points for each one. Multiply by 10 if more than three.

17. How many times have you stopped a course of antibiotics/antidepressants/antipsychotics/heart drugs/or any other vital prescription drugs early and without telling your doctor?

If none award yourself minus 5 points. If once or twice add 0 points; if three times or more, add 2 points for each occasion.

18. Do you have an alcohol problem that you can't control, despite your doctor's best efforts?

If not, count 0 points. If you have been damaged by drink and have really stopped drinking, award yourself minus 20 points (we like patients like this). If you are still drinking too much add 10 points. If you are drunk in the surgery add 200 points. If you show aggression to your medical, nursing or reception staff add 500 points, and don't bother going back.

19. Are you a young parent with children?

Yes? Then give yourself minus 10 points. There's no downside to this question – all GPs know the problems of bringing up kids, and are (I hope) universally sympathetic, regardless of your problems.

20. You are asked to come for your well woman/ man clinic examination. Do you come as asked?

If yes, 0 points. Do you phone in and say the time is inconvenient, but arrange another? If yes, 0 points. Do you not bother and put the appointment card into the wastepaper basket? Add 10 points.

21. How often have you switched doctors over the years, while staying at the same address?

For never or once score 0. For twice or three times score 10. For four times or more score 100.

22. Finally, is your GP's number on your speed dial?

If no, 0 points. If yes, add 10 points, unless you are a young mother, who can be forgiven anything, or someone with a serious illness needing frequent urgent attention.

What is your score?

The dream patient, of course, scores 0 points or even minus points. He or she doesn't exist, but one day I'll meet him or her. I'll ask him/her to marry me, regardless of gender. (It will be a platonic marriage, of course, since I've been their doctor.) You are still a dream if you score 20 points or less. Between 20 and 40 you are the average patient. Don't worry, we still love you. Over 40, and you are entering the 'heart sink' group. More than 60, and you are the sort of patient that drives doctors out of general practice – the true nightmare. If you have scored 300 or more, why do you bother with your doctor at all? It's obvious you don't trust him/her or believe that his/her management of your health has any impact whatsoever.

I made up this scale myself, so it isn't 'validated'. I would like to copyright it, though, as I think it could be a valuable tool for any GP. Were you to fill in this form when you signed up to your doctor's surgery, I'm sure your answers would be very enlightening for the practice, and would determine exactly how the doctor-patient relationship was to progress. I'm happy to offer it to my fellow doctors and wish them good luck with it.

Dr Tom's Top Tips

It's often difficult to know when you really need to see your doctor, or when you can safely treat yourself. So here are my top ten tips for how to deal with common ailments at home, plus the crucial signs that should make you turn to your doctor for help.

Stomach ache

Most of the time it isn't really your stomach but your bowel that's aching – it's full of wind and the bowel wall muscles are going into cramp. Roughly speaking, if the pain is above the navel it's probably stomach, if it's below it's probably large bowel. If it's exactly at the navel, watch over the next few hours to see if it travels down and to the right – that may mean appendicitis.

For upper stomach pains take an antacid: your pharmacist has dozens from which you can choose.

For lower pains, drink plenty of fluids and try to open your bowels. An anti-irritable bowel preparation – peppermint is a good one – may help to relieve the spasm. Peppermint is pretty good for both ends of the gut.

If the pain persists or worsens, then seek advice. That's important particularly if you start to vomit with it, and especially if there's bile in it.

Diarrhoea

This is a sign of infection in the lower bowel. Don't take an anti-diarrhoea medicine. All that will do is prolong the infection: the diarrhoea is your way of getting rid of it. Instead, drink plenty of water to replace the lost fluids, and add salts, sugar and minerals to it. An excellent way to do that is to drink cola – regular though, not the diet kind. If you are near a pharmacy buy some rehydrating sachets. They contain just the right combination of substances to revive the bowel without putting strain on it. Trade names include Rehydrat and Dioralyte and there are others. Take six or eight a day in plenty of water. Avoid rich food and dairy products for 24 hours to give your bowel wall cells a rest. If there's blood in the diarrhoea, see your doctor.

Constipation

What's the best way to get a normal bowel? If constipation is the habit of a lifetime, then you need to change your habits. More variety in your food, with plenty of vegetables and fruit, and drink plenty of water every day, is a start. Believe it or not, physical exercise is a great help. It will help strengthen the muscles in the front of your tummy – your abdominal wall muscles. You need them to be pretty strong to be able to expel a constipated stool.

Don't take laxatives every day. They lead to 'laxative bowel' – a condition whereby the bowels don't actually have the power or the inclination to push the stool further down the path to expulsion.

If you must take a laxative, leave it for a special day, say once or twice a week – no more.

If the constipation is recent, you need to find the cause. A sudden inexplicable change in bowel habit, either to constipation or diarrhoea, in adults, needs investigation. It can be the first sign of bowel or prostate cancer.

Cramp

It is wise to find out the cause, if possible. Muscles go into cramp when their 'electrolyte' or mineral balance is out of kilter. Excessive loss of salt (say, after a day in the sun) or a disturbance of calcium metabolism may be one reason for cramp, although it's often difficult to be sure.

Tonic water (without the gin), which contains quinine, is a classical remedy for cramp, and a glass of it at night may ward off those cramps that wake you in the early hours. Drinking plenty of liquids helps.

To cure cramp, stretch the muscle affected. For example, pull up the foot when you have cramp in the calf, or pull out a toe when it's in the centre of the foot. A lot of back pain is caused by cramp of the big muscles running along the spine: stretch them by arching your back. The best way is to lie on your tummy on the floor, with your hands behind your back and raise both your shoulders and your legs. Do that regularly every day and you may get rid of longstanding back pain.

Can't sleep

Then decide to leave all your daily worries at the bedroom door. Have a snooze radio beside the bed and tune it to a favourite music or talk station – no TV in the bedroom. Don't eat a heavy meal after 8.30 pm, and have only a light warm drink before you go to bed. A warm bath and a comfortable bed are ideal preparations for sleep.

If you really can't sleep after this, talk to your doctor. Sleeping tablets every night are a no-no, as you get used to them. Then not only do they not work, but you get horrendous nights after you stop them. We advise anyone

with sleep problems not to take more than ten tablets in a
month, and never more than on two consecutive nights.

A common cold

That's easy: two or three aspirin or paracetamol three times
a day; plenty of fluids to drink; make a point of resting for
as long as you can each day; and don't go to work in the
first three days. If you do, you will infect everyone else in
your workplace, and that's not fair to them.

There's no antiviral yet for the common cold, so it will
still last for six days, no matter what you do – although you
are only infectious for the first three or four. You will
probably have a hundred colds in your lifetime – every
time a different virus.

Nasty little things, cold viruses.

Infected insect bites

Creams and other applications don't really work, and most
of them only keep the heat of the inflammation in the
skin. Best is to make them as cool as possible.

Put some ice on them for as long as you can tolerate the
cold – say for 10 minutes or so. That will take the heat out
of them and make them less itchy. Re-apply the ice after an
hour or so if the discomfort returns.

An antihistamine tablet once a day (you can buy them

from your pharmacy) may help.

If they get really septic you may need an antibiotic, for which a prescription is needed.

Sunburn

The absolute answer is to cool yourself as fast as possible. So get into the shade and stay there for the rest of the day.

Have a cold bath (a shower may be too painful) and lie in a darkened room with a powerful fan playing on your skin.

If you feel sick, headachy and hot, you have heatstroke, and need to swallow plenty of water, with a generous measure of salt in at least one drink in every four.

Earache in children

Most children get earache at some time, and it is very rarely serious – but the reputation that earache has for being the harbinger of serious disease like meningitis naturally worries parents. A child's dose of paracetamol (trade name Calpol, but there are many other preparations that work as well) is often enough. A cool pack over and behind the ear can also help.

However, warning signs that something more serous is going on are if the child is being sick, complains of a headache, and is tender if pressure is placed on the bone just behind the ear. If any of these symptoms occur, take him or her to the doctor.

Headaches in children

Your child has headaches, and you think he is 'putting them on' to avoid going to school?

You are wrong. Small children don't lie about headaches. If they are complaining, they truly have them. Children get tension headaches and migraines just like adults, but they need to be investigated to rule out other causes.

Only one child in around a thousand who complain of headaches eventually turns out to have a brain tumour, but we can't afford to miss that one case. So children with repeated headaches need to see their doctor.

I'm A Teacher
Get Me Out of Here!
Francis Gilbert

1-904977-02-2 PAPERBACK £6.99

At last, here it is. The book that tells you the unvarnished truth about teaching. By turns hilarious, sobering, and downright horrifying, *I'm a Teacher, Get me Out of Here* contains the sort of information that you won't find in any school prospectus, government advert, or Hollywood film.

In this astonishing memoir, Francis Gilbert candidly describes the remarkable way in which he was trained to be a teacher, his terrifying first lesson and his even more frightening experiences in his first job at Truss comprehensive, one of the worst schools in the country.

Follow Gilbert on his rollercoaster journey through the world that is the English education system; encounter thuggish and charming children, terrible and brilliant teachers; learn about the sinister effects of school inspectors and the teacher's disease of 'controloholism'. Spy on what really goes on behind the closed doors of inner-city schools.

"Gilbert is a natural storyteller. I read this in one jaw-dropping gulp."

Tim Brighouse, Commissioner for London Schools, *TES*

How to be a Bad Birdwatcher
To the greater glory of life
Simon Barnes
1-904977-05-7 Paperback   £7.99

Look out of the window.
See a bird.
Enjoy it.
Congratulations. You are now a bad birdwatcher.

Anyone who has ever gazed up at the sky or stared out of the window knows something about birds. In this funny, inspiring, eye-opening book, Simon Barnes paints a riveting picture of how bird-watching has framed his life and can help us all to a better understanding of our place on this planet.

How to be a bad birdwatcher shows why birdwatching is not the preserve of twitchers, but one of the simplest, cheapest and most rewarding pastimes around.

"A delightful ode to the wild world outside the kitchen window"
Daily Telegraph

Acknowledgements

I couldn't have completed this book without the help and support of a small band of women. First, there is Mandy Little, my agent, who, after a short conversation at a Medical Journalist Association meeting, took me on as a writer. Her faith in me introduced me to Aurea, Vanessa and Emily at Short Books, who have been fantastic colleagues, and whose combined experience of cocktail parties and life in general provided me with a substantial number of the questions (and most of the wackier ones). I must also thank Deanna Wilson, a journalist colleague and good friend for far too many years, for immense help in reading and checking the text, and for a lot of laughs as she did so.

Then there is Lesley Anderson, my artist daughter-in-law, who produced the cover illustration. She has caught the spirit of the book exactly. If you want to see more of her work, then buy my next book, *A Doctor in Collintrae.* Its cover is hers, too, and you will love the cartoons inside.

Finally, I thank my fellow family doctors. This book is for you and your patients. I'm sure that you all could have written it. It's just that I finally had the time to do it myself.

Tom Smith

In case of difficulty in purchasing any Short Books
title through normal channels, please contact
BOOKPOST Tel: 01624 836000
Fax: 01624 837033
email: bookshop@enterprise.net
www.bookpost.co.uk
Please quote ref. 'Short Books'